ANEMIA IN WOMEN

D1565419

IMPORTANT NOTE

The material in this book is intended to provide a review of resources and information related to anemia. Every effort has been made to provide accurate and dependable information. However, professionals in the field may have differing opinions, and change is always taking place. Any of the treatments described herein should be undertaken only under the guidance of a licensed health-care practitioner. The author, editors, and publishers cannot be held responsible for any error, omission, professional disagreement, outdated material, or adverse outcomes that derive from use of any of these treatments or information resources in this book, either in a program of self-care or under the care of a licensed practitioner.

Anemia
IN WOMEN

Self-Help and Treatment

Joan Gomez, M.D.

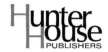

Hunter House Inc., Publishers
PO Box 2914
Alameda CA 94501-0914

Library of Congress Cataloging-in-Publication Data

Gomez, Joan.
Anemia in women : self-help and treatment / Joan Gomez.
    p. cm.
Includes index.
Previously published in 1998 by Sheldon Press in England under the title: How to cope with anaemia.
ISBN 0-89793-366-4 (cloth) — ISBN 0-89793-365-6 (paper)
1. Anemia—Popular works. I. Gomez, Joan. How to cope with anaemia. II. Title.
RC641 .G66 2002
616.1'52'0082—dc21   2001051973

Project Credits

Cover Design: Brian Dittmar Graphic Design

Book Production: Jil Weil/Hunter House

Developmental and Copy Editor: Kelley Blewster

Proofreader: Lee Rappold

Indexer: Nancy D. Peterson

Production Artist: Jil Weil

Acquisitions Editor: Jeanne Brondino

Editor: Alexandra Mummery

Sales and Marketing Coordinator: JoAnne Retzlaff

Publicity Coordinator: Earlita K. Chenault

Customer Service Manager: Christina Sverdrup

Order Fulfillment: Lakdhon Lama

Administrator: Theresa Nelson

Computer Support: Peter Eichelberger

Publisher: Kiran S. Rana

Printed and Bound by Bang Printing, Brainerd, Minnesota
Manufactured in the United States of America

9 8 7 6 5 4 3 2 1   First Edition   02 03 04 05 06

Contents

Introducing Anemia

Anemia is an essentially feminine disorder. Think of the stereotype of a Victorian-era heroine, romantically pale and frail, and fainting at the drop of a bonnet. Among the flesh-and-blood heroines plagued by anemia were that tough cookie Nurse Florence Nightingale, who was bedridden for twenty years due to an unidentified weakness, and the poet Elizabeth Barrett Browning, who spent much of her adult life resting. Elizabeth Barrett Browning suffered simultaneously from another chronic illness—a common situation with anemia—and doubtless both women were made more languorous by their heavy use of laudanum, the heroin of the time.

Anemia is still primarily a female problem today, affecting four times as many women as men, with children coming in second to women. The condition involves a general shortage of blood (*an-* is Greek for *no*; *-emia* means *blood*), the fluid that nourishes and gives life to every cell in every part of the body, from Hillary Clinton's sharp brain cells to Venus Williams's strong tennis arms and shoulders.

The shortage may be in either the quantity or the quality of the blood, or both, but specifically it arises from a lack of hemoglobin, the red, iron-containing pigment in blood that transports oxygen. Royal blood is not immune, as shown by the case in Great Britain of the Queen Mother, hospitalized for anemia a few days before her 101st birthday. Anemia is the most common, most widespread disease in the world, and in 90 percent of victims it is due to a lack of iron, which plays a vital role in hemoglobin's transport of oxygen. It especially affects us women during our golden years from ages fifteen to fifty, when we should be at our healthiest and most productive, and having the most fun—sexually and otherwise.

A high standard of living does not prevent anemia. It is one of the top causes of both physical and psychological ill health among women in the United States, Britain, and Australia—in fact, across all the prosperous regions of the globe. Although poverty is not the direct cause, women in developing countries are even worse off, with anemia affecting virtually all those who are not safely past menopause. This is mainly because of the additional strain of blood loss from parasites in the intestines, common in these regions.

At the most recent count it was estimated that four hundred million women worldwide were running (or more likely walking slowly) on inadequate amounts of hemoglobin. These women are anemic. More than a billion are short of iron—a condition one step away from full anemia.

You would expect that with this constant, universal drain on the health of their citizens from anemia, governments everywhere would be concerned, and would institute advertising campaigns to educate adults and children about anemia—its effects, its treatment, and, most important of all, its prevention. But no such campaigns exist. It seems that anemia is not trendy or sexy enough to excite much interest among politicians, or even among doctors. It does not cause dramatic deaths, but can quietly undermine a woman's health, vitality, and intellectual sparkle for years. It is up to us women to reveal the facts about anemia and to help ourselves.

Common iron-deficiency anemia is one of the few illnesses from which no one need suffer. We know what causes it, it is cheaply and easily avoided or cured, and you don't need a medical degree to understand it. The tragedy is that so many women who are quite severely anemic don't realize it, and they miss out on full health.

Anemia can be easily diagnosed with a blood test—but most people don't ask their doctor to perform a test because they have no idea that they're suffering from a physical illness. Instead, if we feel tired and headachy, get winded running for a bus, and our ability to concentrate is zilch, we women tend to blame ourselves—and then we struggle against nature to do everything as usual, however exhausted we feel.

I was one of these women. For some time—at least several months—I found everything increasingly tiring. I attributed it to my age, nudging fifty, plus a touch of blameworthy laziness. I forced myself to put in more effort. When I had to have a knee operation I was amazed to learn that I was so anemic I would need a blood transfusion before the surgery. It had never occurred to me—a doctor—that I could be anemic. Once I took steps to cure my anemia, I experienced a marvelous, rejuvenating feeling as my body and mind came to life, and I rediscovered the energy and enthusiasm I thought I had lost forever.

HOW DOES SOMEONE BECOME IRON DEFICIENT?

One basic reason our bodies tend to become iron deficient is that we do not intake an adequate quantity of the mineral. The solution to this lies within our power: finding out how to enrich our diets with iron, and applying the knowledge. This does require a little bit of education, for we cannot lunch on a handful of nails, and, disappointingly, we only absorb about 10 percent of the iron in a good, mixed diet and much less than that from such favorite foods as fruits and vegetables (including spinach), eggs, and dairy products.

The other way we become iron deficient is by losing blood, and with it the precious iron contained in blood's red pigment, hemoglobin. This should make it obvious why women are the chief victims of iron deficiency: it is the price we pay for the ability to make babies. To this end, our bodies sustain a monthly loss of blood from the uterus for up to forty years (on average, ages fourteen to fifty-four). Each menstrual period costs 30 milliliters (ml) of blood, containing 15 milligrams (mg) of iron. Since we cannot manufacture iron, this lost iron must be replaced through a bigger dietary intake of it from food or supplements. Added to the regular blood loss may be the huge drain on our bodily resources from building a baby, supplying her with blood while she lives in the uterus, and nourishing her afterwards with the gift of breast milk.

Another cause of blood loss is heavy menstrual periods, sometimes due to the presence of fibroid cysts in the uterus, but often without a clear cause. Nosebleeds or bleeding hemorrhoids are other obvious causes of blood loss, but a slow steady leak from a peptic ulcer, Crohn's disease, or a chest problem can sneakily drip away without either you or your doctor being aware of the situation.

You might think that a woman's diet, compared with a man's, would reflect the fact that she has twice the need for foods that supply iron and protein (hemoglobin is a protein), but the reverse is the case. More often than not it is men who eat the quarter-pounders, who enjoy expensive red meat, liver, anchovies, and other fish—the very foods that best supply iron—while women pass these up and graze on salads and yogurts, good for vitamins but useless for iron. Or we make do with meals of nutritionally empty foods such as bread, cookies, and sweets. How many of us have said, "I won't bother to cook tonight" when it's only ourselves we're responsible for feeding? And it is women, not men, who go on fad diets or deny them-selves, long term, foods they regard as fattening, for instance, red meat and chocolate. Yet these two are among the best sources of absorbable iron.

HOW THIS BOOK CAN HELP

The good news is that anemia—whether from iron deficiency or from one of its other, less common causes—is preventable. *Ane-*

mia in Women: Self-Help and Treatment aims to assist you in identifying the risk factors so you can correct them and avoid the onset of full-blown anemia. But if you've come to this book too late to prevent anemia—if, that is, you've already developed the condition—take heart. As my own history shows, anemia is one health disorder that responds seemingly miraculously to effective treatment. This book, used in partnership with good professional health care, can set you on the best path for regaining your health and vitality.

Read *Anemia in Women* straight through to learn the most you can about the disorder, or treat it as a handbook of sorts, referring as needed to the portions of the text that relate to your situation. Either way, the first and last few chapters offer some good basic information about the topic; they are recommended reading for all women. Chapters 1 and 2 discuss anemia in general and describe the characteristics of your blood, the bodily component upon whose excellent health the prevention of anemia relies. Chapter 3 details the warning signs and symptoms of pre-anemia and anemia. Chapters 4 through 7 each cover specific types of anemia. Chapters 8 through 12 address anemia in the various life stages when a woman is most at risk for it. Finally, Chapters 13 and 14 serve as a health primer with regard to anemia; they outline an anemia-prevention lifestyle, as well as herbal remedies for treatment of the condition.

Anemia is not fashionable; you do not hear people boasting that they've had it. The very word has a Dickensian ring—not surprisingly, since it first came into use in Charles Dickens's lifetime. The Victorians took anemia seriously. The condition is still with us in the twenty-first century, and we, too, should take it seriously. It is time we women staged a quiet revolution and made nourishing ourselves properly a top priority, letting our family come second for once. It is time to be selfish—or sensible.

Chapter

1

Could You Be Anemic?

A SPOT CHECK

For a quick indication of whether you might be anemic, spot-check the following three places on your body: Take a look at the mucous membrane on the inside of your lower lip, gently pull down your lower eyelid and look there, and finally stretch the skin on the palms of your hands so that you can see into the base of your heart line and your life line, the palm's two deepest creases. These three places are always pale in someone who is anemic, even if the person has pink cheeks (pink cheeks can be attributed to a hot room or to the heart pumping the blood fast, for instance after aerobic exercise).

A whole galaxy of possible signs and symptoms of anemia is described in Chapter 3, and if you are anemic you may show one, several, or even possibly none of them. Your hair is a useful giveaway in long-established anemia. Is it becoming thinner, both in quantity and texture? Is it losing its color and going gray if you are dark, or a dirty straw color if you are blond? And is this happening sooner than in your friends or in your mother, if she can remember?

VAGUE SYMPTOMS

Chances are, even if you are anemic, you won't suspect it.

Kirsty said she couldn't have anemia; she ate well, rather too well, and was definitely plump. Her weakness was rolls and buns and bread and potatoes—all of them deficient in iron, vitamins, and protein. Her fatigue was not due to overweight, but rather to anemia from undernourishment.

Carol was slim, in fact verging on anorexic, and she, too, was sure she was not anemic. She ate such "healthy" food— all fruit, salads, and vitamin tablets. She was depriving herself of iron and protein—vital raw materials for making blood.

Susie was losing weight and was trying to live on lettuce, black coffee, and an occasional boiled egg.

All these girls were in the peak age range for developing anemia, fifteen to twenty, and none of them was getting enough iron to reequip her red blood cells as they wore out from daily living.

Eloise felt she was at no risk for anemia. She was forty-one, and she had taken iron tablets since the birth of her one child (she intended to have no more). She always washed them down with her favorite beverage, hot, strong tea. But the tannin in the tea precipitated the iron into insoluble, unabsorbable solids, like the deposit staining the inside of her teapot.

Jennifer, too, felt she could not get anemia because she was taking iron supplements. Quite often, however, she forgot them for several days running, so to make up she would swallow two or three at a time. This was counterproductive. The first tablet would temporarily flood her system with iron, to the point where her body failed to absorb any more.

Most illnesses display overt signals of their presence. You wake up one morning feeling "not quite right," or you are nauseated, feverish, or have a sore throat or pain. You have no doubt that something is wrong when it happens. By contrast, anemia creeps up on you slowly, perhaps taking years, so that you fail to notice the changes as they occur. Besides, the symptoms themselves may be so vague—a fall-off in energy, the stairs seeming steeper, your appetite diminishing for meat meals especially, your memory on the blink—that they're nothing you can identify as "abnormal."

Pre-Anemia

The smart move is to pick up on the situation when you are heading for anemia and zap it while you still have time to sidestep the illness and the challenges of curing it. If your iron level is low and/or falling, you are most likely in a pre-anemic state. Depending on how iron stores are measured, as many as 30 percent of American women of childbearing age are iron deficient (in the same study, the ratio of iron-deficient women increased to 48 percent of those who were regular blood donors); yet only about 5 percent have full-blown anemia. Women who are low in iron during pregnancy are more likely to have a baby that is premature or seriously underweight.

To determine whether you're pre-anemic, one clue to look out for is a reduced capacity for physical work or exercise. For example, I had a patient who became aware she might have a problem because her golf handicap was going up. Or you may first become aware of reduced powers of concentration. This shows up most clearly in schoolchildren, because they are constantly being tested and compared with others.

Iron deficiency—before it reaches the level of anemia—is a health problem in its own right; in fact, epidemiologists label it the world's most common nutrition disorder. Without adequate iron, the component of hemoglobin that is responsible for carrying oxygen cannot be manufactured.

WHEN TO TEST FOR IRON DEFICIENCY

The most useful investigation for determining iron stores is a blood test that measures hemoglobin level; this assessment is always included in routine blood testing. A low hemoglobin level spells anemia for sure. Another method is the serum ferritin test, which measures the concentration of iron in the blood. Some researchers consider it more effective than the hemoglobin test for determining pre-anemic iron deficiency, but it is a more difficult test to perform. Usually the hemoglobin test is enough.

Persons should have their blood tested for iron-deficiency anemia if they fall into any of the following "at-risk" groups for anemia:

* Those undergoing rapid growth, such as during childhood and adolescence, when heavy demands are placed on the body

* Babies under twelve months of age. There is a special risk of decreasing iron reserves between the ages of four months and twelve months

* Those entering puberty, especially during the development of the sex organs

* Pregnant women. Demands are increased by the growing breasts and womb, as well as by the fetus, the placenta, and the amniotic fluid

* Nursing mothers. Although the level of iron in breast milk is small, even a small loss adds up if it is sustained regularly for weeks or months

* Those who have sustained a loss of blood, for example due to surgery or injury. The body requires weeks to make up the loss of blood from a serious injury unless action is taken, usually in the form of a blood transfusion. Meanwhile, anemia makes a patient vulnerable to other illnesses

✦ Women experiencing heavy periods due to the presence
of uterine fibroids or for any other reason

✦ Women who have recently given birth. Blood loss
during childbirth was a common cause of death among
women until Victorian times (this phenomenon is a
rarity today in Western cultures)

✦ Those suffering from bleeding hemorrhoids (the condition thought to be responsible for the Queen Mother's
anemia). Hemorrhoids are easy to ignore if the blood loss
is slight, but can have a serious effect if it is continuous

✦ Persons bleeding from a peptic ulcer or ulcers in the
intestines. The blood shows red if the leak is from low
down in the digestive tract, but may be black if the
blood has traveled far. A black stool shows a substantial
loss of blood from the esophagus or stomach

✦ Persons undergoing long-term use of certain painkillers.
Aspirin and nonsteroidal anti-inflammatory drugs
(NSAIDs), such as ibuprofen, especially can cause bleeding from the stomach. These drugs are used frequently
to treat arthritis

✦ Those who've had a stomach operation, for whatever
reason. Such patients should have an annual blood test
indefinitely

✦ Those who've experienced a loss of blood through the
digestive system due to any other reason. The occult
blood test picks up leaks of blood from the digestive
tract, and is useful when such leaks cannot otherwise
be pinpointed (*occult* means *hidden*)

✦ Persons who suffer from poor absorption of iron and
nutrients—caused by damage to the lining of the small
intestine —because of IBD (inflammatory bowel disorder), ulcerative colitis, or Crohn's disease

↞ Those with bad teeth, who cannot eat meat, nuts, fruits, and vegetables. A diet lacking in these foods is deficient for warding off anemia. A diet composed mainly of soft carbohydrate foods is easy to prepare and swallow, and senior citizens, particularly those who live on their own, often slip into such eating habits

↞ Athletes—amateur or professional—who engage in excessive running and/or jumping. These activities may damage the red blood cells in the feet so that they leak. Some athletes give their hemoglobin a boost with a blood transfusion before a big event, although officially this practice is not allowed

↞ Frequent blood donors, or those who donate when the body's blood reserves are low

Astrid was twenty-three when she took a year off and traveled around South America. In Colombia her money ran out. When she saw a notice offering dollars for blood she thought it would be a simple matter. She had given blood twice before at home in the UK, and had experienced nothing worse than a light-headed feeling for an hour or two afterwards. Giving blood once would have been harmless enough, but she failed to bounce back after a second donation, especially since she was on an iffy diet. She kept experiencing waves of faintness, her energy seemed to have drained away with the blood, and she felt depressed. When Astrid got home a hemoglobin test showed a level of 8 g/dl (grams per deciliter), well below normal (the minimum normal level is 11.5 g/dl for women and 13.5 g/dl for men).

Key Life Stages

As is probably evident from the list above, people are especially susceptible to developing anemia during the following normal life stages. At these times, people need to pay special attention to their diet, and they should undergo blood tests regularly:

+ During the first year of a baby's life

+ During the fast-growing teen years

+ During and after pregnancy, especially while breast-
  feeding

+ While going through menopause

+ In the golden years, over age sixty-five

The special risk factors for anemia in each of these phases in a woman's life are addressed in Chapters 8 through 12.

DANGEROUS DIETS

People who follow faddish or extreme diets are at high risk for anemia—or worse. In particular, the following diets, if strictly followed, provide insufficient nutrition for preventing anemia:

+ The **Zen macrobiotic diet** has ten levels; the "highest" level consists only of grains, with few fluids.

+ The **Beverly Hills weight-reduction diet** consists only of fruit, eaten in a particular order. It cannot sustain the body for long.

+ **Dr. Atkins' diet,** which contains almost no carbohy-drate, has been denounced by much of the medical community as a seriously unbalanced diet. I do not recommend it, although a new edition of his book was introduced in late 2001.

+ **Veganism**—a diet that contains no animal products—can lead to pernicious anemia in particular, with mad-ness and paralysis as severe symptoms. Pernicious ane-mia is caused by a deficiency in vitamin B-12, which comes only from animal products (see Chapters 5 and 6 for more on vitamin B-12 deficiency and pernicious anemia). Breast-fed babies of vegan mothers are at risk of stunted or distorted development.

↞ **Strict vegetarianism** is less dangerous than veganism but can still cause anemia.

ISOBEL'S STORY: A NIGHTMARE WITH A HAPPY ENDING

The whole family was plunged into gloom when Isobel, a sprightly grandmother of seventy-three, fell ill. Even her doctors failed to recognize the cause of her symptoms. She developed odd, jerky movements of her head and arms, would eat hardly anything, and lost weight, but worst of all were the mental symptoms. In the daytime she would laugh or cry at the slightest thing, for instance a picture of a puppy in the newspaper, while at night she moaned incessantly and seemed terrified.

This horror went on for six months. The diagnosis at the time was dementia and the outlook grim. Her husband and children were in despair, until a routine general checkup, which included a blood count, showed that Isobel had less than half the normal level of hemoglobin. Severe anemia was depriving her brain and nervous system, as well as her body, of the oxygen and nourishment it needed to function.

The cure was simple. An immediate transfusion of three pints of blood worked a miracle. Her mind cleared, her appetite returned, and a change in her diet, including the addition of iron supplements, has kept her well ever since. Her hemoglobin level is monitored regularly.

Isobel's was a rare case, and was published in the medical press, but it illustrates dramatically the risk of even very severe anemia being overlooked.

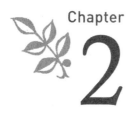

2

All about Your Blood

Blood: It is a sign of danger or violence if you spill it, yet it is the evidence of health in your child's rosy cheeks. It is the very stuff of life. The ancient Hebrews believed that a person's blood contained his soul; this is why the blood is drained off kosher meat. The Romans thought it carried their most esteemed virtue, courage. If a valiant warrior was slain there was competition to drink his blood—and thereby acquire his bravery. Traits of character, good or bad, are still said to be "in the blood," but nowadays the saying has to do with the legacy we've inherited from our parents, that is, the genes.

WHAT BLOOD IS MADE OF

Blood consists of a straw-colored liquid called plasma, which houses three important elements: red corpuscles (*corpuscle* is another word for *cell*), white corpuscles, and myriad minute bodies called platelets.

Red Blood Cells

The red cells—the blood cells that contain life-giving hemoglobin—are the most important ones, but it wasn't until about

1700 that a Dutchman, Jan Swammerdam, first spotted them with his primitive microscope. "Ruddy globules" he called them, but no one was interested. In fact, red blood cells aren't globular but are an unusual shape: like a disc, with the middle part thinner than the edges. This allows them to be squashed into all sorts of shapes without breaking as they are squeezed through the tiniest blood vessels, the capillaries, to carry oxygen to the tissues. If they are the wrong size or shape they cannot function properly, and the person becomes anemic.

A healthy red cell lives for 110 days, give or take three weeks; this means there must be a constant replacement system. (This applies to all the body's other cells, too.)

Francesca's parents came from southern Italy, but they settled in England before she was born because of better job opportunities. Francesca lived a perfectly healthy life until she was twenty-five and got a job as a flight attendant. After a few months she started seeing blood in her urine; this was quite painless, but she became increasingly tired, easily short of breath, and unusually prone to colds and other infections. In spite of a good diet she looked pale and was found to be anemic. Microscopic examination of her blood showed that a number of her red cells were an odd, new-moon shape. These are called sickle cells, and the trait is hereditary. It is most common in Africa, the Arab countries, a few parts of southern Europe, and among African Americans. The sickle-shaped cells tend to get jammed in the blood vessels, and then the white blood cells—the blood's police officers—destroy them. The end result is a shortage of red cells and their hemoglobin: anemia. It was this anemia that made Francesca so tired.

Until she traveled by air regularly her red cells had been, for all practical purposes, normal, and she was not anemic. However, she carried the hereditary sickle-cell trait from her father, which made her red cells vulnerable to the lowering of oxygen levels at high altitudes. They reacted by forming the sickle shape (a similar effect could have occurred if she'd gone under general anesthesia for an operation). Apart from

these situations a carrier of the sickle-cell trait usually expe-
riences no problems and may even be unaware of it.

Francesca could not change her heredity, but she could,
and did, change her job, and meanwhile underwent short-
term treatment for the temporary anemia.

White Blood Cells

White blood cells come in six varieties and are major players in
the body's immune defenses. They fend off bacteria, viruses,
fungi, and parasites that enter the body through the mouth, the
digestive system, the airways, the eyes, and the sexual and urinary apparatus. The white cells are the mobile units of the
defense system, and they are transported in the blood to wher-
ever there is trouble. They spend up to eight hours circulating in
the blood, then four or five days in the affected tissues. Many of
them die in battle with the invading bugs; the resulting debris is
pus. Large numbers of white cells—in addition to steady replacement of the normal reserves—must be produced when there is
an infection to deal with.

Platelets

Platelets are tiny round or oval discs with a life span of two to
three weeks. If a blood vessel is damaged—say, if you've cut your
finger or something worse—a gang of platelets immediately
joins together to plug the hole. With a very small break in the
blood vessel this will be enough to stop the blood from leaking
out; otherwise a clot will form. The platelets play a leading role
in organizing the clotting function. Healing of the wound can
proceed safely when the bleeding has stopped.

Plasma

Plasma is more than just a simple liquid to carry the red and
white cells. It contains 7 percent protein that is available wher-
ever an immediate need exists in the body; usually about fifty
grams a day are required. In states of shock, for instance after a

serious injury or burn, a plasma transfusion can be lifesaving, and plasma is easier to keep and transport than whole blood. An effective artificial plasma also exists. Another function of plasma is to produce antibodies against specific infections (antibodies, along with immunization, serve as long-term defenses both during an illness and in prevention).

WHERE BLOOD CELLS COME FROM

Since none of the vital blood cells are immortal, a constant manufacturing process must occur to maintain supplies. There are urgent calls for extra white cells during infection, and for red cells if the blood becomes anemic from hemorrhage or any other cause—for example, if you move to a city like Quito, Ecuador, where the air is thin due to its high elevation. During the sixteenth-century gold rush to the Andes, the European prospectors became weak and ill, while the native inhabitants remained strong and healthy. The newcomers needed time to produce enough red cells to make the best use of the available oxygen in a new climate.

Unexpectedly, it is ordinary kidney (renal) cells that monitor the supply of oxygen to the tissues all over the body. These cells produce a hormone—a chemical messenger—that triggers the production of red corpuscles. Damage to the kidneys may interfere with this process—one reason why people with chronic kidney disease are always anemic. The control system works both ways: As well as ensuring that there are enough red cells, it also prevents the formation of too many, which could create a dangerous traffic jam in the arteries.

The factory sites for blood-cell production include the bone marrow and—in the unborn baby, up to the fifth month—the liver and the spleen. After that, the liver and spleen begin withdrawing from the task, and the bone marrow takes over entirely. All the bones are involved at birth, but by the age of about twenty only the marrow from the ends of the long bones—the ribs, the vertebrae, and the breastbone—make red blood cells. In an emergency the marrow along the whole leg and arm bone may come back into service temporarily. Older people have less active bone marrow; it may barely cover their needs for new blood. Starvation, for instance caused by anorexia, may also slow down blood production.

THE RAW MATERIALS

Below is a list of vital ingredients for the manufacture of blood. If any of them is in short supply, the body's factories cannot keep up the output required:

+ Iron

+ Protein

+ Vitamin C (ascorbic acid)

+ Vitamin B-12

+ Folic acid

+ Intrinsic factor

+ Vitamin B-6

+ Vitamin E

+ Thyroid hormone

+ Testosterone and other androgens (male hormones— we all have some)

+ Traces of copper, cobalt, and manganese

Iron

Iron—because it is vital in the process of binding oxygen to hemoglobin for transport throughout the body—is by far the most important ingredient in the blood, and it is also the ingredient that people most frequently lack. Large portions of the world's population—such as in India, Thailand, Cambodia, the Middle East, and East Africa—are subject to iron deficiency. In the affluent West, many vegetarians, as well as people who rely primarily on processed carbohydrates for their diet, such as shut-in senior citizens, intake inadequate amounts of iron. Vegans are at particular risk. Diets containing a lot of bread and cereal are high in phytic acid, which prevents the absorption of iron even when it is available. Unfortunately, whole-grain bread and other whole-grain products, which we look upon as healthier than their white-flour counterparts, are more damaging than finely milled white flour in this respect. Similarly, white cane sugar, which is anathema to many health freaks, greatly enhances the uptake of iron.

In the days of King Arthur and his knights, people believed that if you drank wine in which a hero had steeped his sword, you would become strong: the first iron tonic. By the seventeenth century people weren't so romantic. A few rusty nails or iron filings in the wine were found to be just as efficacious. No doubt those who unknowingly were suffering from iron-deficiency anemia did feel better as a result of taking this medicine.

Most of the iron in the body (about 2.5 grams out of a total of 4 grams) is found in the heme molecule, contained in the hemoglobin of the red blood cells (the *hem-* part of *hemoglobin*). Iron deficiency impairs the production of the heme molecule, which is the substance that allows oxygen to bind to hemoglobin and be carried to oxygen-hungry bodily tissues. If you take in more iron than you require, your body simply discards the surplus in the urine. Since hemoglobin is recycled when worn-out red cells are replaced, the body needs only a small amount of iron—about 1 milligram daily—to stay in balance. A small reserve supply, in the form of a protein called *ferritin*, exists in the liver and bone marrow. Myoglobin, another iron-containing pigment like hemoglobin but found in the muscles, is another place where iron is stored. Some iron also circulates in the plasma, but this is reduced during pregnancy unless a supplement is taken.

Iron-containing foods include liver, red meat, dark chocolate, bran cereal, sardines, eggs, and, on the vegetable front, spinach in large quantities.

Protein

Protein is an essential nutrient and is absolutely necessary for making blood. The -globin part of hemoglobin is actually a protein; white blood cells and plasma also contain protein. Dietary protein comes from meat, fish, eggs, poultry, cheese, milk, legumes, and nuts. Proteins from animal sources, including milk, contain all the vital ingredients, or amino acids, for making human protein, but the strictly plant foods, with the exception of soy, do not. That's why it's important for vegetarians to educate themselves about which plant foods contain which amino acids, and to intake adequate amounts of all nine essential amino acids every day. This is especially important in the diets of children, since they cannot grow on a diet of incomplete protein. Nor can the body manufacture blood at any age without high-quality protein. In fact, since making enough hemoglobin is essential to life, this process takes priority over all the body's other protein needs when there is a shortage of protein—including maintenance and building of muscle and organ tissue. This means that inadequate protein in the diet can result in the wasting away of the body's muscles and organs.

Vitamin C (Ascorbic Acid)

Vitamin C is the summertime vitamin; it is found in high quantities in raw vegetables and fresh fruits, with citrus fruits, tomatoes, melons, and berries topping the bill. The Brits were first called Limeys by the Australians because of the limes British sailors ate to ward off scurvy, a disease caused by vitamin C deficiency. Vitamin C improves the absorption of iron. It is found in both the blood corpuscles and the plasma. A shortage causes the red cells to die early and the small blood vessels to leak; the hall-mark of scurvy is bleeding from the gums.

Vitamin B-12 (Cobalamin)

This vitamin is necessary for the maturing of every cell in the body, but especially those in the blood-forming tissues of the bone marrow. It is used in making DNA, the magic double spiral of genetic material that controls every detail of our growth and development. To aid in the development of red blood corpuscles, vitamin B-12 can only work in conjunction with intrinsic factor, a substance made in the stomach.

B-12 is not found in any plant; however, small amounts may be contained on the surface of plant foods from soil residues because B-12 is produced by bacteria. (Much of the B-12 present in fermented vegetable products such as miso and tempeh has been shown to be an inactive B-12 analog rather than the active vitamin.) Not surprisingly, soil residue on your fruits and veggies isn't a reliable source of the vitamin. Therefore, vegans and, to a lesser extent, other vegetarians are at risk for B-12-deficiency anemia and pernicious anemia—the type suffered by playwright George Bernard Shaw—as well as for disturbances of the nerves and a form of madness. Children suffering a vitamin B-12 deficiency fail to grow. Fortunately, the liver stores a two-year supply of B-12, so it takes a long time for a poor diet to produce symptoms. In many cases, even if enough of the vitamin is present in one's diet, he or she cannot absorb it because of a lack of a balance of nutrients.

Foods containing vitamin B-12 include meat, fish, poultry, eggs, and dairy products. Milk is the saving grace for the nearly complete vegetarian, but all vegetarians may be advised to consider supplementation or to consume plenty of foods fortified with B-12.

Folic Acid

Folic acid is among the materials needed to make red blood cells. Although the diet contains plenty of this vitamin under ordinary circumstances, there is a run on it during pregnancy. Pregnant women can become deficient in folic acid—and consequently anemic—if they eat a lot of white bread, white rice, and other refined and processed foods. Natural sources of folic acid include liver, spinach, broccoli, Brussels sprouts, white fish, and whole grains—and, more exotically, oysters.

Intrinsic Factor

Intrinsic factor is made by special cells in the lining of the stomach. It is a necessary substance for the body to absorb vitamin B-12, which enables the red blood cells to grow to maturity and do their work. Chronic stomach disease can interfere with the production of intrinsic factor, and anemia will result.

Vitamin B-6 (Pyridoxine)

This, too, is needed in making hemoglobin. It seldom runs short, because it is present in all types of food: meat, vegetables, bread, and other grains.

Thyroid Hormone

Thyroid hormone promotes the manufacture of all the proteins in the body, including hemoglobin. Too little, as in the condition hypothyroidism, leads to anemia because of slow and limited hemoglobin production. Too much also leads to anemia, because it speeds up metabolism, causing proteins to be broken down as quickly as they are manufactured.

Copper, Cobalt, and Manganese

Just a trace of each of these minerals is needed, and they can be found everywhere. Only in very exceptional circumstances do people suffer a deficiency in any of them.

As you can see, making blood and its prime component, hemoglobin, is more complex than cooking a five-star feast—and the process must be continuous.

HUMAN HEMOGLOBIN FROM TOBACCO?

In 1997 French researchers found a neat way to insert the genes for producing hemoglobin into, of all things, the tobacco plant. The reputation of the deadly weed may be redeemed if it becomes a cheap source of lifesaving hemoglobin, with no risk of contamination by the AIDS virus or any other nasty substance, as exists to a small degree with blood transfusions. Farmers whose livelihood depends on growing tobacco can take heart; even as people—wisely—are smoking less and less, there may yet be a worthwhile market for their crop.

Chapter 3

Symptoms, Signs, and Tests

As we saw in Chapter 1, anemia's early warning system is easily overlooked. The symptoms and signs that should alert someone to the possibility that she is suffering from anemia are deceptively vague. It is easy to think of another reason why you might be feeling washed out, your concentration lapses, or you have had a few headaches recently. And although there are various types of anemia, each with a different cause, the symptoms are much the same in every case. That is because the basic fault in anemia is a shortage of hemoglobin, and the effects of this are the same whatever the cause.

> Angela was forty-one. She had just landed a new job as head nurse in the occupational health unit of the hospital where she worked. It was a major accomplishment, considering the opposition she'd faced, and Angela was enthusiastic to make a good showing from day one. The stimulation of the job interviews had kept her in top form—until now. Now she felt physically and mentally exhausted; she attributed this to the strain she had been under. Another worry—and a major boo-boo—was the fact that she kept getting the name wrong of the nurse who was to be her assistant. She needed to depend on her assistant, and in all probability the woman already felt sore at not having been appointed head nurse herself.

This was not the first time lately that Angela had lost concentration or failed to remember some detail. She felt sure that a good night's sleep would put things right, but that seemed to be the one thing she could not achieve. She no longer needed to worry about getting the job, but still she was unable to relax at night, or indeed during the day, except in a listless, dispirited sort of way. She failed to muster any interest when her eleven-year-old daughter was bubbling over with news about her day at school. And although Angela had the most supportive of husbands, she could not reciprocate. She could not feel concerned about his difficulties at work, or become enthusiastic about sex.

Angela's headaches, located mainly at the front of her skull, weren't spectacular, like migraines, but annoyingly throbbing and persistent. An eye test proved negative. And although she wasn't anxious about anything, at least not at first, Angela kept experiencing palpitations—thumping heartbeats. They were like what happened in a panic attack, but Angela had nothing to panic about. Now and again she felt rather more out of breath than she expected, after running for a bus or climbing a hill and talking at the same time, but she put that down to being out of shape; she hadn't had the energy to go to the gym for ages. Angela wondered if she was becoming neurotic. There was nothing obviously wrong with her physically—unless you counted the minor irritation of two of her nails splitting.

You would never have thought of Angela as anemic. Her face was not noticeably pale. It was the blood test during her obligatory staff medical exam that gave it away. She had iron-deficiency anemia. How could that have happened? As a nurse, she ate a sensible diet, and she hadn't just had a baby. In fact, the underlying cause had been present for years. She had accepted her rather heavy periods as a matter of course since she used an intrauterine contraceptive device (IUD). Anemia makes any bleeding worse, so she had been caught in a vicious circle. Treatment with iron pills brought her hemoglobin up to normal over about eight weeks, and removing the IUD and switching to the contraceptive pill made her periods shorter and lighter.

Since the effects of anemia are so unexpected and general, having just one of the symptoms may mean nothing. But if you have several of the possible symptoms, you should look for signs of the illness, and ask your doctor if he or she thinks a blood test is advisable.

What is the difference between symptoms and signs? *Symptoms* are unusual feelings you experience, such as pins and needles in the fingers, or shortness of breath, and *signs* are what you or your doctor, or even a friend, can actually observe.

SYMPTOMS AND SIGNS OF PRE-ANEMIA

Anemia doesn't suddenly appear out of the blue, except in an emergency situation when a person suddenly loses a lot of blood. There is a precursory, or prodromal, period. It typically develops slowly and exhibits three early warning signs:

* poor exercise tolerance: you can't keep up with the game or the walk like the others, and you don't feel well when you try

* your capacity for work, not only the physical kind, nosedives; you don't get things done the same way you used to

* your concentration wanes before you complete the task at hand; you can't even finish reading a whole chapter

Of course, you may be suffering from a subclinical viral infection, or you may have missed out on sleep lately, but in either of these cases the symptoms pass. With pre-anemia they don't; instead, some of the other symptoms of anemia take over.

SYMPTOMS OF ANEMIA

Lack of energy: you may attribute it to age, or to having your menstrual period or a cold

Getting tired for no reason on more than one occasion: this comes from lacking enough oxygen to fuel the muscles and brain effectively

Shortness of breath: you notice it when going uphill or upstairs or running for a bus, compared with what you used to be able to do. You have to breathe faster to keep the tissues supplied with oxygen since there's less hemoglobin to transport it

Palpitations: your heart beats noticeably harder and faster. Since anemic blood is less efficient at carrying oxygen, the heart has to pump it through the body faster

Throbbing in the head or ears: an effect of the heart's beating harder

Chest pain during exercise: a form of angina. The heart muscle aches like a leg muscle after vigorous exercise. In either case the muscle is complaining that it lacks enough oxygen

Dizziness, faintness: a result of the brain's getting too little hemoglobin and, consequently, too little oxygen

Headaches: also the result of oxygen lack, similar to the effect of being in a hot, airless room

Ringing in the ears: an upset of the nerves and the circulation combine to produce this irritating effect

Pins and needles in the hands and feet: another result of oxygen lack in the nerves

Dimness of vision: a faint darkening of your surroundings, like coming inside out of the sun; again an effect on the nerves, in this case the optic nerves, which convey vision

Poor sleep: you find it difficult to settle down, and you may be restless all night

Poor concentration: an effect on the brain

Low, listless mood: you cannot generate any interest or enthusiasm. This is sometimes mistaken for postpartum depression if it comes on after having a baby, but in the case of anemia it is due to the loss of blood

Sore, uncomfortable tongue: the equivalent of a rash or cracks at the corners of your mouth

Difficulty swallowing: a rare effect, and seen only in iron-deficiency anemia

SIGNS OF ANEMIA

Sometimes it is the *signs* of anemia that first make you wonder if something is wrong, or it may be that you or your doctor look for the signs specifically because of symptoms that have aroused your suspicions.

Pale skin: even if it does not show in your face, particularly if you have dark skin, it may be noticeable in the palms of your hands, or in the color of the nail bed showing through the fingernails. In some types of anemia the pallor has a yellowish tinge

Pale mucous membranes: the special moist skin inside the lips and eyelids. Looking in a mirror, gently pull down the lower lip or eyelid for a spot check

Rapid pulse: a healthy pulse is normally eighty beats a minute or less. The speedup is the result of the heart's having to pump blood faster in order to keep the body's tissues supplied with oxygen

Enlarged heart and/or heart murmurs: both of these are effects your doctor will notice

Swollen ankles: an indication of the heart's having to struggle to do more than usual

Changes in the nails: such as brittleness, ridging, cracking, and a flat appearance. These are signs of iron deficiency and are not seen in other types of anemia

Cracks and soreness at the corners of the mouth: usually caused by a shortage of iron

EMERGENCY SYMPTOMS

If a person loses a lot of blood suddenly, for instance in a traffic accident or from a miscarriage, he or she will experience the following symptoms:

＊ the heart beating faster to prevent blood pressure from plummeting

＊ skin that is pale, cold, and clammy with sweat

＊ the need to lie flat to prevent fainting

An ordinarily healthy adult can afford to lose a pint of blood at any one time without ill effect. This is the amount required from a blood donor. If appreciably more is lost suddenly, the person may go into shock. This is an emergency situation, requiring immediate expert assistance from a paramedic or a doctor. A transfusion of blood, plasma, or plasma substitute can be lifesaving. If a transfusion is not forthcoming, the body will do its best to produce enough plasma to restore the volume of blood over the next twenty-four to thirty-six hours. The subsequent anemia—from the loss of red blood cells—will take at least a few weeks to recover from. If the person has any problems with iron supplies, or if there is another illness in the background, chronic anemia may remain after the acute situation is over.

Chronic Loss of Blood

If someone suffers from, for instance, hemorrhoids, heavy periods, other gynecological problems, or a bleeding stomach ulcer, his or her bone marrow will compensate by increasing the output of new red corpuscles. The extra blood-cell production causes a drain on the raw materials, particularly iron, and iron-deficiency anemia results.

TESTS

If your doctor is on the trail of suspected anemia, he or she may arrange the following investigations:

Preliminary Screening

+ Blood test to measure hemoglobin concentration; packed cell volume (PCV), which is the space in the blood taken up by the red cells; and mean red cell hemoglobin (MCH), which is the average amount of hemoglobin in each
red cell

+ Smear test of blood examined under a microscope, showing the size, shape, and color of the red cells and any abnormalities

General

+ X rays of the chest and digestive system to check for any abnormality that might cause bleeding

+ Occult blood test, to check for hidden blood in the stool

↞ Examination for possible sources of blood loss, including the genital system and fibroids in women, hemorrhoids, peptic ulcer, hiatus hernia, inflammation of the esophagus

Special

↞ Serum ferritin level: more reliable than a simple iron estimation in determining iron-deficiency anemia (ferritin is the storage form of iron in the body)

↞ Serum B-12 estimation

↞ Schilling test: a test for pernicious anemia (this test and the B-12 estimation involve some time and trouble)

↞ Folate level

Laura was nearly sixty, just approaching retirement from her job as secretary at a nearby school. The school had been her life, so it was not surprising that she should feel down as her time there drew to a close. Since her mother had died Laura had lived on her own, which didn't help her spirits. She didn't have the heart to do much cooking for just herself, and anyway, because of a sensitive nature, she had become a vegetarian, almost a vegan. A vegetarian diet was kinder, natural, and less trouble. Besides, if anything, her weight was edging up. She must be eating enough.

As well as feeling "down in the dumps," Laura felt deadly weary and miserably cold all the time, and her voice seemed to be permanently hoarse, although she didn't have a cold. What caught the doctor's eye was her pale, faintly yellowish complexion.

Blood tests showed that Laura was indeed anemic, but not with the common iron-deficiency type. Nor did tests for the vitamins B-12 and folate show the shortage the doctor had expected. In view of her sensitivity to cold and her croaky voice, he decided to do a thyroid check. Laura was suffering from hypothyroidism, an underactive thyroid gland. Because the thyroid gland produces a hormone that is involved in the manufacture of bodily proteins, including hemoglobin, hypothyroidism can be a cause of anemia. Treatment with thyroxine and a review of her diet improved Laura's health and happiness within weeks.

As in Laura's case, when no obvious deficiency or cause of blood loss can be found to account for anemia, a general bodily illness may be the cause. Besides hypothyroidism, disorders of the liver, lungs, and skin, cancers, rheumatoid arthritis, and alcohol excess may all produce anemia as a complication.

4

Iron-Deficiency Anemia

Iron is an essential constituent of the body, totaling four to five grams in the average adult. Most of this is contained in the hemoglobin of the red blood cells, and nearly all the rest is stored in the liver and bone marrow, for making new blood. Some is also stored in myoglobin, a red, iron-containing protein pigment in the muscles that is similar to hemoglobin. The iron contained in hemoglobin, as we have discussed, plays a vital role in the transport of oxygen, which serves as fuel for the body's tissues.

Anemia due to a shortage of iron is a common health problem worldwide. The most likely cause is a loss of blood, including the iron it contains. This problem affects women in particular because of their vulnerable reproductive system. From their first menstrual period, at age twelve and three-quarters, give or take a year or two, women sustain a monthly loss of blood. Then there is the huge demand for blood placed on the body by the fetus during the last half of pregnancy, topped off by a considerable loss of blood during childbirth and delivery of the afterbirth. Men might lose blood from war wounds, especially in the days when doing battle was a more regular occupation, but they do not suffer the inevitable losses that women do just living their normal lives.

Anemia must have always been around, but it was not recognized and named until 150 years ago. However, in Europe starting in the seventeenth century, a condition called *chlorosis* caused concern. It affected adolescent girls and young women, whose complexions became so pale and washed out that they looked faintly greenish (the condition was also called *greensickness*). They suffered from palpitations and became breathless and exhausted at the slightest effort, even climbing stairs, and they had no appetite. Because of their age and sex, their suffering was trivialized and falsely blamed on "lovesickness," but the strengthening medicine generally given at that time—iron filings in wine—seemed to help. Now we know that the sufferers of chlorosis had iron-deficiency anemia.

It was unfortunate that the favorite remedy at that time for almost any ailment, from smallpox to hysteria, was bloodletting. No doubt this was excellent for the overweight, overfed men with high blood pressure, who abounded among the wealthier classes, but it was definitely damaging to an anemic young girl. Other popular treatments included cupping, an alternative method of inducing bleeding, and applying clusters of bloodsucking leeches. Because of a common theory that most illnesses, including chlorosis, were caused by old food going bad in the colon, purging the dietary tract accompanied other treatments, adding to the weakening effect of chlorosis by inducing a loss of protein.

These "cures" remained in use until nearly the end of the nineteenth century. The only sensible idea the doctors had was that diet might be involved in chlorosis. Men ate a lot more than women—especially meat—and they did not suffer from chlorosis. The Victorian miss was told that meat was "too stimulating" for a proper young lady. No wonder so many women died in childbirth, drained of their reserves. Another theory held that tight lacing of the corset caused chlorosis. Loosening the stays may not have helped the anemia, but it must have been a relief.

The breakthrough came in 1895. A Dr. Stockman, from England, recognized that the type of anemia so common in England and on the European continent was due to a shortage of iron. Treatment with iron pills was, and is, rational and effective. Nevertheless, iron-deficiency anemia has not been eradicated. It is endemic among women in large areas of Asia, the Middle East, and East Africa, especially among those who live on unprocessed grain. Even in the affluent West it is still common and often goes unrecognized.

SPOT THE ENEMY: HOW TO DETECT IRON-DEFICIENCY ANEMIA

The general symptoms of anemia are listed in full in Chapter 3. The presence of more than one of those should alert you at once. There are other symptoms to pay attention to as well; these crop up only in cases of iron-deficiency anemia.

Fatigue and Lethargy (How You Feel)

The basic overriding symptom in iron deficiency, as in other forms of anemia, is the extra effort required to get through a normal day. Most sufferers of anemia report a feeling of lassitude before they begin the day and fatigue before they are halfway through. The brain demands a certain amount of oxygen to function well, and if it is short-changed the person feels fuzzy, dizzy, and headachy; she may even faint. Ability to concentrate is zilch. Poor vision can be another problem.

The effect of low-strength blood—that is, blood lacking a sufficient supply of oxygen to adequately fuel all the body's cells—forces the heart to speed up; this can cause palpitations in the chest and throbbing in the head and ears. Second, since the heart gets tired from racing, a sufferer of anemia is likely to get short of breath with any extra exertion, and perhaps experience chest pains, swollen ankles, or ringing in the ears.

Unless a person knows enough to suspect anemia, it isn't the first explanation for these symptoms that comes to mind. Instead, a horrible fear may arise that they have a serious heart or chest disease. The headaches, if they persist, may make the person think they have a brain tumor—and the woolly thinking and loss of concentration may convince them they have early Alzheimer's disease.

> Claire, while studying for her finals, found herself reading the same paragraph over and over and still not absorbing it. Black coffee did not help. Claire decided she was just naturally dim, yet she was at the peak age for anemia, and a hemoglobin test revealed the situation.

Outward Appearances (What You See)

Skin Color

Everyone expects people with anemia to look pale, but skin color can be deceptive. It doesn't depend only on the amount of hemoglobin in the blood. Circulation has a big effect. Even an anemic person can blush, or turn pink with heat or exercise when the blood vessels open up in the skin. But there are two places where it is sometimes possible to see the paleness of the blood itself in someone who's anemic. First, as recommended in Chapter 1, observe the creases in the palms of the hands—the heart line, lifeline, and others. When the palm is stretched wide open these are normally pinker than the surrounding skin; conversely, paleness in the palm's creases indicates anemia. Next, look at the color of the flesh that shows through from underneath the fingernails; in cases of anemia it will be paler than the surrounding skin (this is a particularly useful test for people who have naturally dark skin).

Mucous Membranes

Mucous membranes comprise the moist, delicate lining of the mouth, lips, and eyelids, as well as other parts of the body that are out of sight, such as the inside of the stomach and intestines.

When anemia is due to a lack of iron, the membranes lining the mouth, stomach, and intestines become thinner and more fragile. This may disturb digestion, but more importantly it can prevent the absorption of iron as well as of vitamin B-12. A lack of vitamin B-12 causes another type of anemia, and a person can have both kinds at once.

To investigate for anemia, doctors traditionally spot-check inside a patient's lower eyelid to see if it looks pale, but this test only works if the hemoglobin level in the blood is 9 g/dl or less (the lowest figures regarded as normal are 11.5 g/dl for women and 13.5 g/dl for men, so the eyelid spot check will fail to indicate mild to moderate anemia).

Another effect of iron-deficient anemia on the membranes is the uncomfortable and unsightly symptom of redness, soreness, and cracking at the corners of the mouth, called *angular stomatitis*. It occurs more often in women, particularly in women who wear ill-fitting dentures.

The tongue is often affected by iron-deficiency anemia, especially in senior citizens. The tiny papillae that give the tongue its rough appearance all but disappear, leaving the surface looking oddly bald. There may be one or two deep fissures, but they don't hurt, and patients can still taste food properly.

Fingernails and Hair

Nails are particularly sensitive to a shortage of iron. The first symptom often noticed by sufferers of anemia is brittle nails that split and crack at the edges. Sometimes there are ridges running toward the tips that tend to split. At the next stage, the whole nail becomes flat instead of curving to the shape of the finger, and it looks curiously dry and dead. Finally, a condition called *koilonychia* (literally, *spoon-shaped*) may develop, wherein the nail becomes concave instead of convex. The nails provide a measure of how much iron there is in the body as a whole, by analysis of the clippings. A total of less than four micrograms (mcg) per gram of nail constitutes deficiency.

Like the nails, the hair is a special, insensitive outgrowth from the skin. In iron-deficiency anemia the hairs become thinner and break more easily.

Difficulty Swallowing

Some patients with iron-deficiency anemia complain that they feel "something in the way" when they swallow. This symptom is uncommon and affects mainly middle-aged women. It is caused by a thin web of tissue partially blocking the esophagus just below the larynx (voice box), and is part of the general upset to the lining membranes. It has two names, because doctors found the condition so interesting that they wanted their own names attached to it. It is called the *Plummer-Vinson syndrome* or the *Patterson-Kelly syndrome*. It never completely prevents swallowing and recovers with the rest of the anemia.

Disturbed Vision

In very severe iron-deficiency anemia, particularly if it has come on rapidly, for instance with a loss of blood from exceptionally heavy periods, small hemorrhages may occur in the retina at the back of the eyeball; these are visible to the doctor during an eye exam. This is a rare occurrence and is treated with lasers.

Geraldine was sixty-nine. Upon her retirement as a biology instructor at a women's college, she had taken up several new interests, including involvement in a local literary group, a hospital volunteer organization, and the Natural History Society. Even with all her new pastimes, she was slowing down and seemed to get tired at the slightest exertion. Still, she would have told you that she was perfectly well, thank you, but of course you couldn't expect to stay young forever. And she had endured a lot of dental trouble lately. She wore dentures, and the lower set in particular was slipping around in her mouth, making it awkward to eat properly. If she was with other people she certainly could not risk eating anything with seeds or that needed chewing, so she tended to stick to soup, mashed potatoes, hot cereals, and cake. At home she dunked her cookies in tea. None of these foods provided her with iron. To make matters worse, she had developed sore places at the corners of her mouth, little raw cracks that made it uncomfortable to open her mouth very wide. She did not feel it was right to bother the doctor with something so trivial. Nor did she think it justifiable to mention the tingling she had been getting in her fingers lately. It was like the feeling you get when you warm your hands by the fire if they've gone dead with cold.

Then Geraldine started experiencing difficulty swallowing, and she became truly frightened. She was sure, immediately, that it was cancer. She imagined a tumor swelling in her throat and choking her. She could feel something in her esophagus, just below her voice box. She paid a rare visit to the doctor, who seemed concerned and interested and examined her thoroughly. The physician could see nothing abnormal at the back of Geraldine's throat, but she noticed her poor color. Both her skin and the insides of her lower eyelids were unusually pale. Her pulse rate, 95 beats per minute, was unduly fast, considering that she had been sitting chatting with the doctor for ten minutes. The doctor also thought she could detect a hint of swelling around Geraldine's ankles.

The physician arranged a routine blood test and a barium swallow. For the latter, Geraldine went to the hospital, where she had to drink a glass of thick, white, pepperminty liquid while they did an X ray. The two reports came back just over a week later, and Geraldine, with her scientific training, was eager to see them and have them explained.

Geraldine's physician told her that she had severe iron-deficiency anemia, and that her sore mouth, lack of zest, and the swallowing problem were all part of it. The blood test was the evidence:

Hb (hemoglobin): 8.1 g/dl
(normal for a woman is 13.5–15.5 g/dl)

RBC (red blood corpuscles): 4.1 millions per ml
(normal is 3.9–5.6 millions per ml)

PCV (packed cell volume): 26.8 percent
(normal is 36–48 percent)

MCV (mean corpuscular volume): 65 fl (normal is 86–95 fl)

MCH (mean corpuscular hemoglobin): 19.6 pg
(normal is 27–34 pg)

These results showed that Geraldine's blood was deficient in hemoglobin, although she had a normal number of red cells. The proportion of her blood comprising cells in relation to the fluid plasma (PCV) was well below normal, because her red cells were undersized (MCV). Each red cell also contained less hemoglobin than normal (MCH), even allowing for their small size.

This picture of small red cells containing too little hemoglobin is typical of iron-deficiency anemia. (Since the iron in the blood is nearly all contained in the hemoglobin, there was no need in Geraldine's case to do a separate estimation of the iron content of her blood.) A blood smear confirmed the situation, showing the small, pale cells, some of them oval and other odd shapes.

The barium-swallow X ray showed that a fragile web of lining tissue was interfering with the free passage of food down the gullet (esophagus), the appearance typical of Plummer-Vinson syndrome. This is an uncommon complication of iron-deficiency anemia, so Geraldine's physician referred her to a consultant hematologist, a specialist in blood disorders. Her treatment was begun with an iron injection, followed by the standard iron-supplement tablets.

ANEMIA IN CHILDREN

Babies

An anemic mother starts her baby at a disadvantage, so the doctor's order to take an iron supplement during pregnancy is really important to follow. Babies need a high level of hemoglobin—and iron—when they enter the big world, since they readily become anemic, whether fed by breast or by formula. They are especially vulnerable if they start life at a small size or premature, or if their introduction to a mixed diet is delayed much after the age of four months. Even the very best milk is inadequate for providing iron. Weaning foods should include pureed meat and green vegetables, plus orange juice, which helps the absorption of iron. Indications that a baby is short of iron include an undue lack of activity, poor appetite, a quiet whininess, and a failure to hit his target weight. The pediatrician will notice the problem and suggest the best treatment.

Older Children

Older children, too, may become anemic. Their reaction is seldom what you would expect. Rather than sitting quietly, looking sorry for themselves, they are likely to get in trouble at school for being inattentive, show no motivation for work, and wear everyone out by being hyperactive. They also tend to catch any illness that is around. An anemic child will lack the intellectual liveliness that most children exhibit, even though he has a perfectly good brain. This is because his brain is starved of the generous supplies of oxygen needed in increasing quantities up to age twenty.

Badly behaved children always should be regarded with suspicion that an illness exists underneath the mischief. One curious habit that may arise in iron-deficiency anemia and be mistaken for naughtiness is called *pica*. It comprises eating inappropriate substances like coal, sand, or a diet of nothing but peanuts.

> Jessica, age six, was the bane of her mother's and her teachers' lives. She was always into something naughty or dangerous, seemed incapable of sitting still for five minutes, and made no progress at school. She wasn't interested on the one hand, and on the other, she didn't remember what she had been told from one minute to the next. It was partly due, her teachers thought, to her missing so much school. It seemed

as though she always had a runny nose or a cough. Her resistance to infection was poor, and her appetite was pathetic.

Jessica's granny told her that she would never grow big and strong enough to be a ballet dancer if she didn't eat her healthy meat and greens—but Jessica just didn't feel hungry. An odd thing—which made her mother take her to the doctor yet again—was that she had found her eating dirt, cramming it into her mouth as though it were food. The doctor explained that this was pica. It can happen in children with severe learning difficulties or in pregnant women, but Jessica was neither. It doesn't always involve eating something as weird as dirt or coal or wood, but instead may appear as an exaggerated craze for a particular food, such as peanuts or eggs. Children who are short of calcium have been known to eat the plaster off the wall, but those deprived of sufficient iron may eat almost anything unusual. Adults with iron deficiency can develop pica, too.

Alice, a perfectly sensible woman of fifty, had an overwhelming desire for carrots; she ate so many that her skin developed a slightly orange hue and her general nutrition suffered. She, like Jessica, had iron-deficient anemia. Iron replacement cured Alice of this peculiar symptom, and in Jessica's case her transformation into a normal, pretty little girl was a slow miracle.

TESTS

With any of these signs or symptoms, it is essential to consult your doctor, who can order some definitive tests, such as the following:

- Blood count, to check hemoglobin level and the state of the red blood cells

- Smear test, to assess the look of the red cells in particular; by looking at the cells, a hematologist can recognize blood disorders as easily as you can recognize a friend's face

✦ Radio-iron test, to determine if iron is being absorbed properly

✦ Serum iron estimation, to check if the blood contains the normal amount of iron

✦ Urinary iron, to see if too much is being lost by this route

✦ Occult (means *hidden*) blood test, to determine if blood is being lost from the digestive tract

✦ X ray of chest and neck, in case there are lung or thyroid problems

CAUSES OF IRON-DEFICIENCY ANEMIA

The three most common causes of iron-deficiency anemia are:

✦ Loss of blood, which automatically means loss of iron

✦ Inadequate diet

✦ Malabsorption

Any of these is more serious if it arises at one of the stages in life when a person is naturally particularly vulnerable: from age four months to twelve months; as a fast-growing adolescent; during pregnancy and childbirth; and, to a mild extent, for all premenopausal woman. In later life the bone marrow doesn't have the resilience to quickly make up for any blood lost, so that, too, is a vulnerable period. (See Chapter 1 for a more detailed exploration of at-risk groups.)

Loss of Blood

By far the most common cause of iron-deficiency anemia is loss of blood, with its valuable content of iron-containing hemoglobin. Although the body carefully recycles the hemoglobin from the worn-out blood cells that have come to the end of their life, it can do nothing about blood that is actually spilled or red cells that break inside the blood vessels. The iron in hemoglobin is more difficult to replace than the protein in hemoglobin, which the body can make up from its internal resources. The iron reserve in the bone marrow is quickly used up when there is an extra call on it to make new blood.

Menstruation

Some blood losses are normal for women. Take an ordinary menstrual period: A woman loses a total of 20 to 40 mg of iron each month. This means that, throughout the month, all year, a woman needs to take in and absorb at least 2 mg of iron daily, instead of the daily 1 to 1.5 mg required by men, children, and those past menopause. Paradoxically, if a woman is anemic already, she tends to lose even more blood than usual with each period.

Pregnancy, Childbirth, and Breast-Feeding

Having a baby is normal, too, but it places a dramatic drain on the mother's iron supplies, especially starting in the twenty-fourth week of pregnancy. All in all the baby-to-be demands between 400 and 500 mg of iron during the course of the entire pregnancy. This averages out at double the mother's usual requirement over the nine months, despite her having no periods. You can see the urgent need for taking iron pills during this time (see Chapter 10 for more about avoiding anemia in pregnancy).

The birth, including delivery of the blood-rich afterbirth, depletes the mother's iron reserves of another 300 mg, and possibly much more if it is a difficult birth.

Breast-feeding drains iron supplies as well. It calls for an extra 0.5 mg of iron daily, over and above the basic requirement, which depends on when the menstrual periods start again.

Blood Donation

If you donate two pints of blood during the year, you must absorb an extra 1 mg of iron daily throughout the twelve months. You cannot replace the iron as quickly as you can give it away.

Heavy Exercise

Joggers and competition runners are healthy, but 50 percent experience a temporary anemia. Probably all that is needed is to make sure they're eating a well-balanced diet.

> Amy and Tim were among the happiest couples you could imagine—until the twins came. Amy had been an only child and always said that she would make sure to have "a real family" with four children, two boys and two girls. They lived on the outskirts of a country town, ideal for children, and Tim commuted to his job in the city. Money wasn't flowing, but there was enough. There was no financial reason to avoid putting their plan into operation. By ages twenty-four and twenty-eight respectively, Amy and Tim had their four children. Tim junior was four, Edward two and a half, and the twins, identical girls, were fifteen months.
>
> Amy hired a helper who took a lot of the physical chores off her shoulders, and Tim pulled his weight on weekends. But Amy couldn't enjoy her little ones or anything else about her life. She was unreasonable with the helper and edgy with Tim, sex had essentially disappeared from her life, and nothing seemed worth the bother. Amy had lost her appetite and her hair was a mess, with no spring or shine. The world, as she saw it, seemed tinged with gray.
>
> Amy was anemic. She had taken her iron and folic-acid supplements religiously during the pregnancies, but that hadn't been enough. The four babies had come too close together, and the final straw was having twins. Each over six pounds at birth, they had drained Amy's iron stores—and to cap it all off, she decided to try breast-feeding them. Six weeks of this exhausted her completely and she was forced to give up. Amy's doctor gave her one iron injection, prescribed tablets for a whole year, and ordered strict instructions to have no more babies without getting a blood test first!

Other Causes

Sudden, severe blood loss may occur if you are unlucky enough to be involved in a terrible automobile or industrial accident. A varicose vein may bleed alarmingly after a trivial bump; you may have a miscarriage; or you may experience heavy bleeding around the time of menopause. These are emergency situations, requiring urgent medical or paramedical attention. They will also necessitate follow-up treatment with iron supplements for many months to restore the lost blood and the health that goes with it.

Chronic blood loss is by far the most common and most often neglected reason for the development of iron-deficiency anemia. This is because the bleeding is likely to be so slight that it is ignored or goes unrecognized, although it takes the loss of only a teaspoonful of blood daily to cause anemia over time (since the body is not able to restore quite as much iron as it loses).

The area most prone to silent bleeding is the digestive tract, from mouth to anus. Bleeding gums can occur at one end, or hemorrhoids, internal or external, at the other. The swallowing tube (esophagus) can become inflamed and ooze blood as food passes down it, particularly if a hiatus hernia is impeding the food's progress into the stomach, which has a tougher lining than the esophagus. The pleasantly warm sensation when brandy or other strong drink goes down is an indication of its irritating the lining membrane en route. Heavy drinkers tend to develop varicose veins in the esophagus; these are much more delicate than varices elsewhere. A serious hemorrhage can result from trivial damage.

Similarly, if the stomach or duodenum becomes ulcerated, perhaps due to the helicobacter bug's settling in this area, a slight but continuous loss of blood may result. Even more likely, and probably the most common cause of iron-deficiency anemia in some Western countries, is bleeding in the stomach caused by irritation to the lining from painkillers such as aspirin or the anti-inflammatories (NSAIDs), which are often used to treat arthritis and rheumatic pain. There may be stomach pain as well as bleeding; this can be alleviated to some extent by adding another medicine, misoprostol.

Steroid medication, used in asthma and other illnesses, can have a similar effect on the stomach. The bleeding will not be enough to make a noticeable difference in the color of the stool, but enough to cause anemia.

An occult blood test will detect traces of altered blood in the stools and is a standard investigation for anemia. It will, of course, also pick up evidence of bleeding lower down the digestive tract, for instance from polyps in the colon, a cancerous tumor, or the common, age-related condition of diverticulosis. Diverticulosis is the presence of small pouches in the walls of the colon; the pouches tend to get inflamed and to bleed a little.

Women's reproductive organs readily bleed for a variety of reasons—from psychological stress to fibroids or a cervical erosion. Chest disorders may lead to a loss of blood from coughing. Much blood can be lost from a nosebleed, and kidney and bladder disorders may produce blood in the urine. All these different problems can lead to iron-deficiency anemia from external blood loss.

Another major cause of deficiency of usable hemoglobin is *hemolysis*: bleeding inside the blood vessels themselves due to breaks in the surface of the red blood cells. The hemoglobin thus released into the fluid part of the blood is lost to the body since it passes out in the urine, a condition called *hemoglobinuria*.

There are various causes of hemolysis, including:

✦ incompatible blood transfusion

✦ certain drugs and medicines

✦ severe burns

✦ some snake and spider bites

✦ malaria, tuberculosis, liver disease, and some hereditary blood disorders

All these things can cause iron-deficiency anemia because loss of hemoglobin means a disproportionate loss of iron, but for 99 percent of us it is simple bleeding—for instance from heavy periods, or because of antiarthritic medication—that is at the root of this problem.

Inadequate Diet

If you eat an ordinary mix of foods, you probably take in 15–20 mg of iron every day, but you only absorb about one-tenth of this. Men need 1 mg daily; premenopausal women need a little more, since they lose blood with periods. Since we lose about 1 mg a day in the skin we shed, this is a tight balance. It seems necessary to have much more iron available in the diet than we actually absorb and retain.

The prosperity we enjoy in Western developed nations does not automatically ensure a diet adequate in iron. In certain parts of the UK, for example, the amount of iron in the average diet is seriously inadequate, and is reflected in very low hemoglobin levels among the people living in those areas. This is largely a matter of diet: too many refined carbohydrates in the form of cereal, buns, potatoes, scones, and biscuits; too little meat and fresh greens. The best foods for providing iron include liver, red meat, sardines, and bran cereal; but you must beware of unrefined cereals and grains, for they contain phytates, which inhibit the absorption of iron. Vitamin C enhances iron absorption; so eating plenty of vitamin C–rich fruits and vegetables is also important.

Malabsorption

Even if you eat foods containing iron, certain factors can inhibit the body's absorption of the iron. For starters, not all iron in foods is created equal in terms of its bioavailability, that is, how readily it is absorbed by the human body. The iron from animal-based foods, called *heme iron*, has a greater bioavailability than the iron from plant-based foods, called *nonheme iron*.

Additionally, certain naturally occurring substances present in the food itself can prevent the absorption of iron. Phytic acid, or phytates, found in grains and eggs, are naturally occurring substances that prevent the proper absorption of iron. The tannin in coffee and black tea, as well as in alkali medicines used for indigestion, has a similar effect. These substances act by forming an insoluble compound with the iron so that it cannot dissolve in the blood and body fluids; it is like putting a stone into a drink instead of a lump of sugar. Vitamin C in large quantities reverses this effect, and white sugar also helps.

TREATMENT

The treatment of this common disease is cheap and easy: You need to take iron supplements. You might think going "the natural way," by changing to a diet rich in iron, would be better. Unfortunately, while a good diet may *prevent* anemia, once a person has the disorder it is too late. This is because anemia involves a vicious circle: The more anemic one is, the more easily she bleeds, for instance during menstrual periods, and the smaller her appetite. The most effective form of iron in supplements is the salt iron sulfate; a dose of 200 mg (the normal pill size) provides 67 mg of pure iron. To recover from anemia a person needs to take one of these pills three times a day.

You may wonder why you can't take the full day's supply all at once. If you take the iron with or after a meal, it isn't absorbed as well as when the stomach is empty, and even then there is a limit to how much the stomach can deal with at any one time. The next snag is that once the stomach has received a dose of iron, it refuses to accept any more for about six hours. So the total dosage needs to be spread over three separate occasions,

and preferably be taken before meals. While recovering from anemia, people need to avoid phytic-containing whole grains and
brown rice and to eat no more than one egg a week; instead, to
get the most benefit from the pills, they should choose white
bread, white sugar, and plenty of vitamin C.

> *Important note:* Be aware that small children are at deadly risk
> if they take adult iron tablets by mouth. For children, liquid prepa-
> rations are available, and also some chewable tablets for toddlers
> and older children up to about ages ten to thirteen, depending on
> the weight of the child.

The beneficial effects of iron supplementation will begin to
show after about two weeks; the doctor will monitor the
patient's progress with blood tests as the hemoglobin level gradually rises. If the hemoglobin level fails to rise, it is an indication
that the anemia's underlying cause is still present. When hemoglobin has reached a normal level, the patient must continue
with the treatment for a further three to six months to replen-
ish iron stores.

Side Effects

All this sounds easy in theory, but many people have problems
taking iron; they experience stomach pains, diarrhea, gas, or constipation. Unfortunately, the slow-release preparations, aimed at
bypassing the stomach, are less efficacious, because the iron is
released too far down in the intestinal tract for absorption.
Other iron salts, such as ferrous fumarate and ferrous gluconate,
are less upsetting to the stomach than iron sulfate, but they provide only half as much iron so they must be taken over a longer
period of time.

Another option for avoiding the unpleasant effects often
caused by conventional iron tablets is to obtain supplemental
iron via herbal medicines; see Chapter 14 for more on this topic.

Iron Injections

For some people, oral iron supplements simply don't work. Their anemia may be severe enough—for example, during late pregnancy or following major surgery—that supplements alone are ineffective. And a few unlucky people find it impossible to take iron by mouth because of stomach pain, vomiting, and diarrhea. For these groups, injections are the sole remaining option.

Iron injections are usually given once a day into muscle tissue, with the dosage carefully calculated according to the person's size. Too much is poisonous, and iron going into a vein instead of a muscle is dangerous.

Blood Transfusion

Blood transfusion is an immediate treatment for severe anemia, but it runs the risk of throwing a strain on the heart in a severely anemic person.

Iron Overload

Transfusion, iron injections, or even taking iron supplements for too long without a blood test can cause iron overload. This can also occur in people with alcoholic cirrhosis or who drink a lot of cheap red wine or certain beers, and among the Bantus in Africa, who do all their cooking in big iron pots. Too much iron causes liver problems, but a little extra does no harm. While it is a mistake to go on taking iron supplements indefinitely, for instance after fully recovering from pregnancy-related anemia, it makes good sense to stick to the preventive diet long term.

Chapter

5

Anemia Due to Shortage of Vitamin B-12

It was not until 1948 that cobalamin—vitamin B-12—was isolated, and several years after that when its vital role in the production of hemoglobin was discovered. This led to the recognition of anemia due to B-12 deficiency. B-12 is not found in any fruit or vegetable; therefore, unless the vitamin is taken in the form of supplements or fortified foods, some animal products are an essential part of the human diet. (Plant foods can contain B-12 on their surface from soil residues, but this is not a reliable source of the vitamin.) Vegetarians are obviously at risk of becoming deficient in vitamin B-12, and vegans, who avoid all animal products, even eggs and milk, are certain to run out of the vitamin as their stores are used up. For them, especially, regular supplementation with B-12 is vital.

Smoking of any tobacco product—cigarettes, cigars, or pipes—depletes the body of vitamin B-12. This is because tobacco smoke contains cyanide, and the vitamin is used by the body to detoxify this substance. Most of us can easily afford to draw on our reserves for this purpose, but not a vegan.

Another, apparently innocent circumstance can contribute to B-12 anemia: a gross imbalance between the intake of vitamin

B-12 and that of folate (folic acid), another of the B-complex vitamins. Normally these two vitamins act in combination as an essential step in making blood. B-12 is found only in food from animal sources, and folate comes mainly from plants. If B-12 is in short supply in the body, too much folate is dangerous. It uses up the scanty B-12, with especially damaging effects on the nervous system. Fruit, vegetables, and nuts, so often recommended as "healthy," are all loaded with folate but devoid of B-12.

SYMPTOMS AND SIGNS OF B-12 DEFICIENCY

A person entering the early stages of B-12 deficiency won't exhibit all the possible symptoms. The trick is to be alert to any single one of them, and if it persists over several weeks, to have it checked out.

The symptoms of B-12 deficiency include:

+ Any of the general symptoms of anemia (see Chapter 3). As with all forms of anemia, some of its effects, such as poor sleep and easy fatigue, may tend to be written off as resulting from worry, the weather, or age

+ A beefy-red, sore tongue—often the first sign of the illness. It is worse when eating hot foods or those with sharp flavors. The inflammation comes and goes, regardless of attempted treatment with diet, lifestyle, or drugs

+ Alternatively, an unnaturally smooth and pale tongue

+ Soreness and cracks at the corners of the mouth. These are far less common than in iron-deficiency anemia

+ Pale skin and membranes, which, as the anemia becomes more severe, take on a lemony tint, including the whites of the eyes. This is because the red blood cells fail to develop properly and tend to leak hemoglobin into the plasma. There, hemoglobin's red color changes to yellow.

The anemic person may fail to notice the change in her own appearance; a friend whom she hasn't seen for ages or a new doctor may be the first to draw her attention to it

↞ Darkening of the urine. This is an occasional secondary effect

↞ In a few cases, a darkening of the skin with the natural pigment melanin, a symptom more noticeable in fair-skinned Caucasians. The reason for this effect is unknown

↞ Bruises appearing mysteriously, often on the thighs or arms

↞ Occasional, unexplained diarrhea, with no relation to what the person has eaten

↞ Changes in the blood leading to clotting in a vein, or blockage in an artery, with serious local symptoms including pain and swelling, paralysis, or death

↞ Heart problems. If the anemia comes on so gradually that the patient fails to notice anything unusual, the first indication of trouble may be the beginnings of slow, congestive heart failure. The person feels short of breath following any effort, his ankles may swell, and he has no energy

↞ Infertility—a possibility to bear in mind if another cause of infertility remains undiagnosed

↞ Possible serious effects on the unborn child of a woman short of B-12 during pregnancy. However, B-12 deficiency during pregnancy is very rare in the West; it crops up in cases of dire poverty, as in some developing countries, or as a result of a really weird diet (e.g., consisting of peanuts only, fruit only, or other odd combinations lacking balance). The worst effect on the developing fetus is spina bifida, but cleft lip or cleft palate may also result

✦ An unexpected inability to throw off an infection. This may be the first symptom of a slowly developing but severe lack of B-12. The blood-making arrangements in the bone marrow become so out of kilter that they cannot produce the components of the body's defense system

Symptoms Involving the Brain and Nervous System

A large group of symptoms involving the nervous system and brain affect some people suffering from vitamin B-12 deficiency. These include:

✦ Pins and needles, burning or tingling, or numbness and cold, usually starting in the feet and later involving the hands. These sensations affect both the right and the left sides equally; they usher in the nervous symptoms of the illness in 80 percent of cases. It may not at first occur to the doctor that these could be the result of a vitamin-deficiency syndrome

✦ "Glove and stocking" anesthesia: a loss of sensation in the hands and feet. The person may lose joint sense as well, which especially makes control of the legs difficult

✦ Difficulty maintaining balance when walking, so that the person easily trips and falls

✦ Muscular weakness and stiffness, most troublesome in the legs. The sufferer tends to drag his toes as he walks

✦ Blurring of vision. The optic nerve, which serves eyesight, may be damaged by a lack of B-12

✦ Muddled thinking, forgetfulness, lack of usual interest and initiative. This can shade into dementia over time, if left uncorrected

The symptoms of B-12 deficiency showing up in the nervous system only occur in a minority of cases; as a group they are called, rather alarmingly, *subacute combined degeneration of the cord*. The cord referred to is the spinal cord, the big column of nerves running inside the backbone, connecting the nerves between the limbs and the brain. Sometimes the nervous system reacts to a lack of vitamin B-12 before anemia sets in, but the cause and the cure are the same.

Although pins and needles are most often the first symptom of this complex of symptoms, any of them may occur first, including the intellectual fuzziness. This symptom may fail to be recognized until the patient begins to recover. Then, as mental alertness returns with treatment, he realizes that he had not been himself mentally for many months. The victims of these types of mental symptoms are nearly always the elderly, and more often men. Nevertheless, neither men nor women of any age are immune.

> Judith, for example, was only thirty-three when she began to lose her intellectual edge in her high-powered sales job. Once her problem was accurately diagnosed as B-12 deficiency and treatment begun, she made a complete recovery.
>
> Agnes, on the other hand, was more typical. She was seventy-three, had worked in a government office until age sixty, and had four children. After she retired she continued working as a crossing guard at the nearby elementary school. She boasted that she had never had a day's illness except for a bit of trouble with her bowels now and then. Agnes fell into low spirits when she was told she must give up the crossing job, which she loved, because her eyesight was no longer good enough.
>
> After that she seemed to go downhill. She became increasingly forgetful—she who had prided himself on knowing the names of all the children who passed through her intersection—and she lost her enthusiasm for life. She couldn't even bother to follow her favorite soap operas. And another thing:

Her walking had definitely grown unsteady, and she'd had one or two nasty falls; they shake you up at age seventy-three.

Neither Agnes nor her family thought it was unusual for someone her age to be a trifle vague and to stumble occasionally. A case of old age, the physician had said reassuringly and advised Agnes to put her feet up and take it easy. After all, she was well past retirement age.

It was a doctor filling in for Agnes's regular doctor while he was on holiday who decided to explore different possibilities that might perk Agnes up. The new doctor had examined her with a fresh eye, unlike her family doctor, who was lulled by familiarity into thinking that she seemed the same as she always had, only a little older. Agnes's blood tests showed that she was severely anemic and that her serum B-12 was alarmingly low. The injections he gave her worked a miracle. Her mental capacity returned, and she regained her sure footing.

In Agnes's case it had not been a matter of poor diet but rather a bowel problem that had led to her anemia. With Judith it had been the aftermath of a business trip to Japan, where she'd eaten a raw fish dish. For more about these causes, and others, keep reading.

CAUSES OF B-12 DEFICIENCY

One or a combination of the following causes can lead to a deficiency in vitamin B-12:

+ Following a vegan or other diet grossly deficient in animal products

+ Consuming an excess of dietary folates. Folic-acid supplements or an excess of folates in the diet can tip the balance of vitamin B-12 and folate by using up an already scanty supply of vitamin B-12

+ Overgrowth of bacteria in the intestine. This can occur in diverticular disease, a wear-and-tear effect in which

little out-pouchings develop along the intestinal wall.
Germs normally found in the bowel can "hide" in these
little pouches and multiply to a greater number than
normal. This may cause loose bowels and discomfort,
but these symptoms may only be very slight. A larger
problem occurs when the bacteria prevent the intestine
from absorbing the usual amount of B-12. That is what
happened to Agnes. Treatment with tetracycline controls the infection

⁺ Crohn's disease. Crohn's, which affects the small intestine more often than the large, is a serious condition
that impairs absorption of B-12 (and other nutrients).
Sometimes it causes a fistula or passageway to form
between two loops of gut; a section of intestine is thus
bypassed and becomes a breeding ground for germs

⁺ Celiac disease. This condition usually appears before age
two, but it occasionally goes recognized until adulthood. It involves a congenital lack of the enzymes that
enable absorption of ordinary foodstuffs, for instance
wheat products. Vitamin B-12 is poorly absorbed, too.
Affected children fail to thrive; affected adults are
slightly anemic and vaguely ill

⁺ Stomach operations or chronic gastritis. These conditions also disturb absorption and often lead to pernicious anemia (see Chapter 6 for more on pernicious
anemia)

⁺ Certain parasites. The fish tapeworm, for instance,
which is present in raw fish, can deplete all of the available vitamin B-12; this is what happened to Judith.
Meat from fish-eating animals in Scandinavia and Asia
can also introduce the tapeworms. Effective medicines
for treatment include niclo-samide and praziquantel;
thorough cooking of the fish or meat is the best prevention for tapeworms

+ Diabetic diarrhea. Diabetes sometimes upsets the nerves controlling the muscles of the intestines, resulting in constipation or watery diarrhea, typically at nighttime. In this situation, B-12 cannot be absorbed and anemia develops

+ Certain medicines that interfere with the absorption of vitamin B-12. These include neomycin, an antifungal used in some skin and ear problems; and metformin (Glucophage), used in diabetes

+ Stagnant-loop syndrome. The body's twenty-two feet of intestine lie in closely packed coils and loops in the abdomen. As long as the partly digested food travels down the intestine at a steady rate, squeezed along by the intestinal muscles, no problems arise. Bacteria are always present in the gut; they play an essential role in breaking down the food for digestion and absorption. The muscular movement can become sluggish under the influence of several types of medicine, including painkillers, tranquilizers, sleeping pills, and antidepressants, and in the senior years a general slowdown occurs. In these circumstances a loop of gut may miss out from the general flow—a so-called stagnant or blind loop—resulting in a buildup of material where bacteria multiplies, sometimes up to two or three times their normal numbers. This results in bouts of colicky pain and loose stools, which may be pale and fatty or sometimes dark with blood, and in the intestine's loss of ability to do its job of absorbing all the proteins, fats, carbohydrates, and vitamin B-12 needed. Two special types of X ray clinch the diagnosis: a barium swallow and a barium enema. These involve taking in, by mouth or anus, a liquid that contains barium, which shows up on the film and gives a picture of any abnormality in the gut. If some anatomical quirk exists at the root of the problem, a surgical tidy-up is required, but in most cases tetracycline, a bacteriostatic medicine, controls the excess of bacteria. The dosage is 1–2 grams daily. After three or four days of treatment, vitamin B-12 and other nutrients will start to be absorbed properly. If the underlying condition seems likely to continue, a seven- to ten-day course of tetracycline should be taken every six months, indefinitely.

TESTS

If a diagnosis of B-12 anemia is suspected, some combination of the following tests will be performed:

+ Blood tests will show a very low hemoglobin level and a reduced number of red cells.

+ Chemical test will show a reduced serum B-12 level.

+ Blood film will show oversized and/or oddly shaped red cells.

+ Other screening tests (to check for other causes of this blood picture) include liver function, thyroid function, and the Schilling test (see page 31). These three tests will yield normal results if the problem is purely a lack of B-12.

TREATMENT

Emergency

Patients with a very low hemoglobin level—less than 4 g/dl— need a blood transfusion. Specifically, they need a concentration of red blood cells, given slowly so as not to throw a strain on the heart by suddenly expecting it to pump an extra quantity of blood. Frusemide, a diuretic (which rids the body of excess water), is given for the same reason: to reduce the volume of fluid in the body.

Standard

Treatment in less acute cases of B-12 anemia consists of injections of hydroxocobalamin (vitamin B-12). One thousand micrograms is injected twice a day for one week, then once a week for the next six weeks, and after that four times a year for life. If the B-12 anemia arose from an inadequate diet, an appropriately altered diet plus an injection once a year should provide healthy quantities of the vitamin to the body.

The bone marrow swings into full production within forty-eight hours of the first dose of B-12, and normal, healthy red cells begin flooding the bloodstream days after that. All this production of hemoglobin-filled red cells may use up the person's reserves of iron, so his or her doctor may prescribe a course of iron supplements, starting soon after the injections have begun. (A patient's blood film will show extra-pale red cells when he or she is short of iron.)

> Helen was fifty-nine, warmhearted, and comfortably plump. Her three grandchildren loved visiting her; one of the highlights of their visits was tea, when Helen served her scrumptious homemade cakes and cookies. Her diabetes was a nuisance, but she refused to let it spoil everything. It had developed about four years ago, just after her husband suffered a heart attack. The doctor said hers was a quite mild case of adult-onset diabetes, and that she should be able to control it by diet alone. This very quickly proved impossible.
>
> It wasn't that Helen ate a lot, but she liked the wrong things: cakes and scones and cornflakes, plus vegetables, including potatoes (French fries were her favorite), and the apple a day that was supposed to keep the doctor away. She wasn't a great one for meat, especially since her husband had died; it was just easier not to cook since she was by herself now. Her new dentures did not help, either.

In the end Helen's doctor prescribed Glucophage, an antidiabetic medication. With that, and doing the best she could to manage her diet, Helen's diabetes came into reasonable balance. She continued taking the Glucophage, and for a few years never noticed any side effects. Lately, however, she had been feeling increasingly tired and listless, partly, perhaps, because she'd had a run of minor infections. It was only a small thing, but her feet were like two blocks of ice and her fingers often went dead even when the weather wasn't particularly cold. Then there was that big purple bruise that had appeared as if by magic—she couldn't remember bumping herself. But what was more troublesome was getting so winded at the slightest exertion, and sometimes feeling slightly nauseous.

When she went for her next routine visit to have her diabetes checked, Helen mentioned getting short of breath and feeling generally under par. The doctor gave her a thorough examination, including an electrocardiogram (for her heart) and a blood test. The tests revealed that Helen was severely anemic, and having to pump the poor-quality blood through her body at an increased rate put a strain on her heart. Her anemia was caused by a shortage of vitamin B-12. Her diet was not ideal, but the basic cause of Helen's anemia was the Glucophage, one of the drugs that may, in some people, prevent the body from using the B-12 in their food. The low level of Helen's B-12 stores indicated that the deficiency had taken two or three years to build up.

With rest, heart tablets, B-12 injections, and, later, iron supplements, Helen eventually recovered completely, but it took a long time. The Glucophage, the villain in the situation, was replaced with a different antidiabetic medication, and for the sake of her heart as well as her diabetes, she managed to reduce her weight.

Chapter 6

Pernicious Anemia

Pernicious anemia (also called *Addisonian anemia*) is a very special form of anemia associated with a deficiency of vitamin B-12. It is more important than the others, because it accounts for 80 percent of the sufferers of B-12-deficiency anemia, and until halfway through the twentieth century it was invariably fatal. It is also more mysterious than the other B-12-deficiency anemias. It is not due to any shortage of the vitamin in the diet, nor to malabsorption.

In 1849 Dr. Thomas Addison of Guy's Hospital in London first described a group of his patients with this illness. It had nothing to do with a lack of iron, the only known cause of anemia at the time, and all the victims died. It was feared as much as cancer is today. Although the disease was named after him and he was desperate to help the victims, Dr. Addison found no cure.

The breakthrough did not come until 1926. Two Americans from Massachusetts, Doctors Minot and Murphy, found that eating large quantities of raw liver every day kept their pernicious-anemia patients alive and well. We know now that this was because of the vitamin B-12 stored in the livers of the animals, but no one had even heard of this vitamin until after the Second World War.

A Dr. William Castle attended a lecture by Dr. Minot—and came away intrigued. There was obviously something in liver that anemic patients needed; since the substance came from outside the body, he called it *extrinsic factor*. But since ordinary people don't need vast quantities of liver to stay fit, he reckoned that something was lacking in the bodies of the anemic patients themselves. He labeled this substance *intrinsic factor*, and he tracked it down to the gastric juice, the digestive juice produced in the stomach. Even when his patients had eaten plenty of liver and were apparently well, Dr. Castle found that their gastric juice was different from normal; however, seventy years ago no technology existed to analyze gastric juice.

He found that if he regurgitated the contents of his own healthy stomach and administered this to his pernicious-anemia patients, they felt much better—even without eating all that liver. (Presumably he did not spell out to them where he had obtained the "new medicine"!) Since he could not provide an ongoing supply of his own gastric juices, the patients had to continue eating liver, but at least their illness was now better understood. In due course concentrated liver extract was manufactured and then produced in an injectable form, so the treatment became less unpleasant. The second breakthrough came in 1948 when, simultaneously in Britain and America, vitamin B-12, or cobalamin, was isolated (and identified as the extrinsic factor Castle had speculated about); a few years later it became available as an injection. No one today dies of pernicious anemia, and no one need even feel poorly because of it.

CAUSES OF PERNICIOUS ANEMIA

The underlying cause of pernicious anemia is a lack of usable vitamin B-12 in the body, created by the absence of intrinsic factor in the gastric juice. (Intrinsic factor in a healthy individual facilitates absorption of vitamin B-12.) The lack of intrinsic factor in some people comes about from an autoimmune reaction.

Pernicious anemia is one of a group of autoimmune diseases, in which the body's defense system turns against some of its own cells, in this case the gastric parietal cells (the cells of the stomach wall). If any of your blood relatives has an autoimmune disorder, you are more likely to get one or more of them yourself.

Another autoimmune disease that often occurs in those with pernicious anemia is vitiligo, a condition wherein the skin loses its brown pigment, melanin, in patches that show up dead white. Otherwise, the skin remains perfectly smooth and healthy and feels no different from usual. The white patches can occur anywhere on the face and body, and the condition gradually spreads. It seems worse in the summer because, as the rest of the skin tans with the sun, the areas with vitiligo remain obstinately pale. Makeup is useful for hiding the condition on the face.

CHARACTERISTICS OF THE PERNICIOUS-ANEMIA SUFFERER

Pernicious anemia occurs more often in people who meet the following characteristics:

* People of northern European descent. It can affect people of any race, anywhere, but it is rare in the tropics and especially common in northern Europe. Even so, it affects only one in ten thousand people

* Blue-eyed people more than brown-eyed people

* Those with a tendency toward prematurely gray hair

* Women more often than men, in a ratio of three to two

* Ages forty-five to sixty-five, with a peak at sixty. It is unusual in those under thirty

* Those with blood type A

Other autoimmune disorders likely to crop up in pernicious-anemia patients or their relatives include:

✦ vitiligo (see above)

✦ diabetes

✦ rheumatoid arthritis

✦ underactive thyroid (Hashimoto type)

✦ overactive thyroid

✦ systemic lupus erythematosus (SLE)

✦ certain liver diseases

✦ dermatomyositis

SIGNS AND SYMPTOMS

Pernicious anemia is an illness that comes on slowly and gently, with symptoms and signs that don't ring immediate alarm bells, so sufferers may fail to realize the urgency of the need for treatment. Without adequate treatment, however, victims are headed toward disaster, with the loss of their physical health, sanity, and, finally, life.

All the signs and symptoms of pernicious anemia result from a deficiency of usable vitamin B-12; therefore, they are the same as the signs and symptoms detailed in the preceding chapter. Also review the general symptoms of all anemias, listed in Chapter 3.

Pay particular attention to the following:

✦ Pallor, with a faint lemon-yellow tint, including in the whites of the eyes

✦ Occasionally a darkening of the whole skin, especially noticeable in the skin folds

- A pale and smooth tongue, sometimes sore, red, and inflamed

- Pins and needles in the feet and hands

- Weight loss, with no obvious change in appearance

- Difficulties with memory and concentration, or virtually any psychological symptoms, from panic attacks to mild dementia

- Deadly fatigue, as in all types of anemia, but likely to be particularly severe. This is because pernicious anemia is apt to become well advanced before the illness is recognized

- Tendency to bleed unduly, for instance from heavy periods, nosebleeds, etc. This is a sign that the blood factory in the bone marrow is so desperately short of B-12 that the platelets, which aid clotting, are not being produced in adequate numbers

TESTS

Tests run by a doctor when investigating for pernicious anemia will include the following:

- Blood film will show unusually large red corpuscles; instead of round they will be oval and other odd shapes.

- Hemoglobin test will indicate a low or very low level.

- Red-cell count will be low.

- Serum iron level will be high.

- Serum B-12 level will be very low.

Only in Pernicious Anemia

Certain signs will show up only in pernicious anemia:

⁌ Presence of anti-intrinsic-factor antibodies in the blood (in up to 50 percent of cases). These indicate that the body is fighting against the production of intrinsic factor

⁌ Lack of the normal stomach acid

⁌ Abnormal Schilling test. This occurs when a dose of vitamin B-12 by mouth is not properly absorbed unless intrinsic factor is given as well (in ordinary B-12 deficiency, adding the intrinsic factor makes no difference, since the vitamin is absorbed anyway)

Edith had been a glamour girl at nineteen, a blue-eyed honey blonde, and her appearance was just as important to her at sixty-nine. She belonged to the generation that came of age before having a suntan became fashionable, and so she stayed out of the ultraviolet rays. Since she was proud of her pale skin, she did not mind that it seemed to be getting even paler. She explained away the yellowish tinge with something she'd read about blondes having olive undertones to their complexion. If olive, why not yellow? On the other hand, she had been disappointed when her hair had lost every vestige of color by the time she was fifty. Now, in her late sixties, her snow-white coiffeur looked elegant.

Then the vitiligo started. Patches of really white skin appeared and spread, making the remaining pale skin look unattractively muddy and yellowish by comparison. The notion of leprosy came to Edith's mind, but the doctor assured her that what she had was perfectly harmless. Edith informed him that otherwise she was quite well. She had been fortunate with her health for most of her life, although she was sad to have had no children. She and her ex-husband had certainly tried.

Finally, Edith's legs started letting her down. She'd experienced the odd tingling sensation in her feet for years, but now she found herself walking rather unsteadily. Particularly when it was dark, she liked to find a rail to hang onto. When the practice that Edith's physician belonged to offered all their senior patients a general checkup she decided to go along. Ordinarily she did not like to bother her doctor. He might think she was fussing about nothing if she complained about such things as feeling tired, not sleeping too well, and forgetting what she had done with her keys. But this was an open invitation.

The nurse who was doing the screening got worried when she saw Edith; she asked the doctor to have a look. After he had examined Edith he told her she was anemic and arranged some tests. These showed that Edith had a very low hemoglobin level (6 g/dl), big oval red cells, and a positive Schilling test. She had severe pernicious anemia and required treatment urgently. The condition must have been building up for years, the doctor said, to have gotten so bad; it might even have affected her inability to have a baby. That in turn had been a factor in her divorce.

When the doctor asked her about autoimmune illnesses in her family, Edith remembered an aunt, years ago, who had a thyroid problem and might have been anemic; but, of course, that had seemed irrelevant to Edith's own health.

The specialist whom her doctor brought in decided that, because Edith's hemoglobin was so low, her treatment should start with a blood transfusion. The effect was immediate. She felt as though life itself had been introduced into her veins; and when this was followed by the first few weeks of B-12 injections, Edith felt—and looked—ten years younger, stronger, and happier.

LOOK-ALIKE ANEMIA

People who have part of their stomach surgically removed—for instance, to treat an ulcer or some other stomach problem—run a 50 percent risk of developing a syndrome just like pernicious anemia, characterized by shortages of usable vitamin B-12 and intrinsic factor. This is because the cells lining the stomach, which make the intrinsic factor and the stomach acid, have been removed.

A lesser procedure called *vagotomy* involves cutting a nerve to the stomach to switch off the production of acid. The problem is that this also cuts off the production of intrinsic factor, resulting in symptoms that look like pernicious anemia.

The treatment for this look-alike condition is the same as for pernicious anemia.

TREATMENT

Treatment options for pernicious anemia are similar to those for anemia from B-12 deficiency.

Blood transfusion is a lifesaver in any very severe anemia; but see Chapter 5 for precautions related to giving blood transfusions.

After the blood transfusion, or for less severe cases of pernicious anemia, the patient will receive **injections** of hydroxocobalamin (vitamin B-12) into a big muscle. The standard regimen calls for injections of 1,000 micrograms, given twice in the first week, then once a week for six weeks, then two to four times a year (with tests to assess progress) for the rest of one's life.

How the Injections Work

Ordinarily, vitamin B-12 (extrinsic factor), which is contained in some foods (for instance meat), comes into contact with the intrinsic factor in the stomach. The two factors are made for each other and immediately join together. The combination travels down many feet of small intestine until it reaches a special place located just before the entrance to the colon, or large intestine. There the two factors uncouple, the vitamin is absorbed into the bloodstream to be used by the body, and the intrinsic factor is discarded with the waste products.

The reason the two factors combine temporarily is to save the vitamin B-12 from being digested with the rest of the food, until it reaches the safe area at the end of the small intestine. If a person lacks intrinsic factor—because of autoimmune antibodies or surgery—it is useless to give him or her B-12 by mouth, because the vitamin will be destroyed by the digestive juices. Injections into muscle tissue bypass that difficulty. The body can store B-12 for quite a while, so once levels are built back up to the healthy range, only occasional "booster shots" are needed. An injection two or three times a year is a small price to pay for normal health—especially compared with eating half a pound of raw liver every single day!

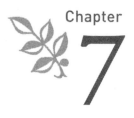

7

Other Types of Anemia

By the 1930s doctors knew about the common anemia caused by lack of iron, and about the far more dangerous pernicious anemia that could be kept in check by something in raw liver that we now know to be vitamin B-12. Lucy Wills, a pioneering doctor working in Bombay in 1931, was distressed at the number of pregnant women there who became ill. They were generally in poor health and exhausted, and instead of gaining weight they tended to lose it—a worrisome situation in pregnancy. These mothers were anemic, and they often died during childbirth because of the inevitable loss of blood. Iron tonics failed to help them, and anyway their symptoms—for instance, pins and needles in the hands and/or feet, or an inflamed tongue—were more reminiscent of pernicious anemia. Also, under the microscope, their blood films showed big, oval red cells, not the little round ones of iron deficiency. Eating liver did not help, so Wills guessed these women must be lacking something else.

She considered their diet: mainly rice or bread with very little meat or vegetables. She tried giving the same food to monkeys—and they too became weak and weary like Wills's patients. After trying all the foods she could think of, Wills hit on one that cured the problem: yeast extract (Marmite). She did not know about folate, or folic acid, a B-complex vitamin yet to be discovered, which was the factor in yeast that cured her patients.

FOLATE-DEFICIENCY ANEMIA

Folates work in conjunction with vitamin B-12 to enable the body to make DNA, the essential blueprint for the production of all new cells. Since red blood cells have a strictly limited life, and because they are the most numerous of all the cells in the body, anything that inhibits cell production affects them the most. Inadequate cell production leads to a type of anemia with a reduced number of red cells, many of which are the wrong size and shape. A shortage of either vitamin B-12 or folate produces these effects, and the symptoms and signs and appearance of the blood film are similar to each other.

CAUSES OF FOLATE DEFICIENCY

Diet

Folates are found in some meats and to a lesser extent in raw vegetables. A diet based on bread, rice, pasta, or overcooked food is likely to be short on folates. Strict vegetarians, including vegans and people who eat a vegetarian diet for religious reasons, such as Hindus and the Indian populations of South Africa and Fiji, are all at high risk for developing folate-deficiency problems. Babies fed exclusively on goat's milk will be short of folate, whereas cow's milk or human milk contains just enough of the vitamin for their needs.

In the United States, Britain, and other Western countries, the only people likely to have a diet deficient in folates are the old, the poor, and the housebound, who may tend to exist on bread, buns, and cookies, with a little cereal and milk. Additionally, people who adopt a faddish diet may miss out on folic acid. A low- or no-folate diet will have an effect on the blood within days.

Pregnancy

The developing fetus places a tremendous drain on the mother's reserves of B-12 and folic acid. Her body's B-12 store is ample to see her through pregnancy and the puerperium (the period between childbirth and the return of the uterus to its normal size), but her folate store is quickly used up. In the first twelve weeks of pregnancy many women feel nauseous and eat very little, especially meat and vegetables, yet these are vital weeks in the baby's development. In fact, to avoid all possible danger of serious congenital disorders in the baby's nervous system, women trying to get pregnant are advised to start taking supplements of folic acid even before they conceive! At the very latest women should begin supplementing with folic acid as soon as they suspect they are pregnant. It is not only in early pregnancy that folate is important. In the last half of the pregnancy the baby is growing so fast that he needs a big, steady supply of folic acid—and everything else. (See Chapter 10 for a discussion of nutritional needs during pregnancy.)

Physical Illness

Any illness, especially if it involves inflammation, calls for extra supplies of folate for the repair work. Examples include tuberculosis, malaria, skin diseases such as eczema, dermatitis with peeling, Crohn's disease of the intestine, and all forms of liver disorder. But stagnant-loop syndrome, so troublesome for B-12 deficiency (see pages 59–60), actually causes an increase in folate levels. The bacteria trapped in the blind loop can manufacture folates.

Celiac disease particularly causes problems in folate metabolism, and it is always associated with a lack of folate. The basic problem in this disorder is an inability to digest gluten, a component of wheat; secondarily, the absorption of folate is hampered. Celiac disease may take a year or more to show. It usually arises before age two; in such cases the child is obviously ill and the doctor will be involved. If the illness, including lack of folate, develops later in childhood, the youngster's growth is held back and puberty is delayed. In other cases the syndrome is not diagnosed until adult life, although it is likely to have been present for some years, but with symptoms too mild to arouse concern. The usual adult symptoms are diarrhea, loss of weight, and anemia, but some elderly patients don't experience the diarrhea.

Natasha was sixteen and only four feet eight inches tall when her mother started to worry seriously. Her daughter seemed to be a girl Peter Pan: Her body was still a sexless child's shape with only the tiniest breast buds and almost no pubic hair. She had not started her periods. The final trigger that made Natasha agree to see the doctor was the soreness and blistering that broke out on her forearms. The doctor said it looked like dermatitis herpetiformis, which is fairly common in celiac disease, so he asked a few pertinent questions. Natasha did not suffer from diarrhea, but she was a fussy eater. Although she was underweight her abdomen bulged out more than one would expect. She was very pale and felt generally under par. Investigations with a specialist confirmed the family doctor's provisional diagnosis: celiac disease with profound folate-deficiency anemia.

Treatment of the celiac disease and supplements of folic acid helped Natasha to grow and develop, although she never quite caught up in height. The dermatitis settled down within a few weeks of beginning the treatment.

Alcohol

Alcohol drunk regularly in substantial quantities is a potent cause of folate deficiency, and sometimes also of iron deficiency. Fifty percent of heavy drinkers are anemic, although they may be unaware of their condition. Hard liquor is especially harmful, while beer has the redeeming feature of containing folates.

The reasons for folate deficiency in heavy drinkers include:

↞ a direct toxic effect of alcohol on the bone marrow, interfering with blood production

✦ a chronic loss of blood from the digestive tract, which is liable to become inflamed and to ulcerate anywhere from the esophagus to the anus

✦ a bleeding tendency that is part of the alcoholic syndrome, especially in people with cirrhosis

✦ an inability, present in any liver disorder, to properly metabolize B-12 and folic acid. Such a condition allows B-12 to build up, but the folate is washed out with the waste

A further disadvantage of alcohol is that it increases the chances of having antifolate drug reactions. The diuretic (water tablet) triamterene, which is normally free of side effects, is one such drug that can produce problems with folate absorption in heavy drinkers. The inhibitory effect on folates of some other drugs is also made worse by alcohol; see the section titled "Antifolate Drugs," below.

Anyone on a junk-food diet or any diet that doesn't provide enough folate will begin to show signs of folate-deficiency anemia in about nineteen weeks. If alcohol is added to the inadequate diet, the deficiency shows up within two weeks.

Kirsty worked in the high-stress world of advertising, and at thirty-three she earned an income that paid for a flat in an exclusive neighborhood and a silver Mercedes. Her wretchedly heavy menstrual periods, which were getting worse, didn't fit her image of keeping everything under control, but the symptom that finally sent her to the doctor was a rash. Apart from her propensity for big bruises—"You only have to look at me and I get a bruise," she complained—she had crops of small flat spots all over her body and limbs. They started off bright red and then changed to purple, finally fading into a brownish-yellow—and then a new lot would appear. Her doctor said this was called purpura; it wasn't an illness, but a reaction. He inquired into her general health.

Kirsty had to admit that she had lost energy and concentration lately, and even her social life was suffering. Although she felt tired, she couldn't sleep, and an alcoholic nightcap didn't help. Tests showed that Kirsty was anemic, with big red cells and a shortage of platelets in her blood film, and a deficiency of folate in the serum. The cause was tracked to her alcohol intake; she admitted she tried to keep pace with the men, and a good Scotch whisky was her drink of choice. Treatment to boost her folates would be useless unless she called a halt to her drinking for several months; even then, any return to drinking would have to be on a very moderate scale. Wine would be better than whisky, if she really felt the need to drink something alcoholic.

The good news: In most cases of alcohol-induced folate deficiency there are signs of recovery within a few days of stopping drinking. In particular, the lack of platelets is speedily reversed. Platelets are the tiny blood cells that are essential for clotting. Especially in cirrhosis or an acute liver upset, the platelet count plummets, and hemorrhages, small or large, result. A lack of platelets was the cause of Kirsty's heavy menstrual periods, her easy bruising, and her purpura.

Kidney Disease

Particularly if the person is on a hemodialysis machine, folates tend to be washed out of the body in the urine. The situation is a little better with peritoneal dialysis, but folate supplements must be taken in any case.

Heart Disorders

The congestive type of heart trouble makes the liver congested also, and this in turn leads to a loss of folate in the urine.

Underactive Thyroid

Underactive thyroid (hypothyroidism) can be a direct cause of folate deficiency.

Hemolytic Anemia

Hemolytic anemias, those in which the red blood cells are destroyed, as in sickle-cell anemia, can lead to a shortage of folate as well as of other vital constituents for making blood.

Antifolate Drugs

Some medicines can prevent the body from taking up folate, although this response doesn't always happen. They include:

- The antiepileptics phenytoin, phenobarbital, and primodone. These cause folate depletion so often that supplements of the vitamin are given with them routinely

- The antibiotic trimethoprim (Septrin, Bactrim). It is most likely to cause trouble when it is taken long term as a preventive, for instance for recurrent bladder infections

- Sulfasalazine, used in diseases of the intestines, for instance Crohn's disease, which itself leads to folate and B-12 deficiency

- Pyrimethamine (Daraprim), an antimalarial

- Triamterene, a diuretic (see above)

SYMPTOMS

Folate-deficiency anemia reveals itself in ways similar to B-12 deficiency and pernicious anemia, detailed in Chapters 5 and 6, respectively, as well as to the general symptoms of anemia, listed in Chapter 3.

To recap a few of these, watch for:

- an inescapable feeling of lassitude

- pale skin, lips, and eyelids, sometimes tinged with a lemon color

- shortness of breath with effort

* heart palpitations

* dizziness

* thoughts and ideas less clearly focused

* a sore tongue

* occasional diarrhea

* mild fever at times

* a tendency to lose weight

In folate-deficiency anemia the sufferers are likely to be much younger than those with pernicious anemia or simple B-12 deficiency. On the whole the symptoms are less severe, and only a minority of patients develop a sore red tongue.

TESTS

Lab tests will yield the following results in cases of folate-deficiency anemia:

* Serum folate: low

* Red blood corpuscle folate: low

* Serum B-12: normal, or may be high

* Blood film: big oval cells and some misshapen ones, as in B-12 deficiency

The doctor will also perform a test to assess dietary folate intake, and a biopsy of the duodenum to check for celiac disease.

TREATMENT

Unlike treatment for B-12 deficiency, including pernicious anemia, which involves getting B-12 injections for life, a person can absorb folic acid from tablets taken by mouth; some doctors even suggest that a cure by diet alone might succeed. However, most people want to get better as soon as possible, and oral supplements achieve this.

There is one constraint. An excess of folate over B-12 in the body can use up the B-12 to such an extent that serious neurological and mental problems are likely to develop. Except in pregnancy, when vitamin B-12 is usually present in ample supply (and probably being monitored by the doctor), before starting folate treatment it is essential to test the level of B-12 in the serum and make sure it is not depleted. A booster B-12 injection can be given if necessary.

The usual regime consists of one tablet containing 5 mg folic acid daily for four months, only continuing if the underlying cause of folate lack has not been found and dealt with. In severe sickle-cell or other hemolytic anemias, one 5-mg tablet weekly is a precaution against a dip in folate level. In the hemolytic anemias so much new blood is required to make up for the blood cells lost that a person can run short of folate (and other nutrients). While taking the folic acid supplements, and continuing afterwards, a diet rich in folates makes good sense. This involves eating salads and raw vegetables whenever possible, and some meat, preferably beef. A list of the folic-acid content in certain foods is included below.

PREVENTING FOLATE DEFICIENCY IN PREGNANCY

Several methods are utilized for preventing folic-acid deficiency in pregnant women and their babies:

- ✦ Daily doses of 400–600 mcg (micrograms) of folic acid during pregnancy. Larger doses might lead to a relative lack of vitamin B-12, resulting in symptoms in the nervous system or brain of both baby and mother. Because there is a tendency for pregnant women to run short of iron, most prenatal folate tablets also contain iron. Any

side effects from the combined tablets, such as stomach
pain and either constipation or diarrhea, will be due to
the iron; therefore, a folic-acid-only tablet is available

↞ Folic-acid supplementation in women who might
become pregnant. Serious abnormalities, preventable
by the mother's taking folic acid, can develop in the
unborn baby in the early days of pregnancy, so supplementation should be started as soon as practicable—
ideally in the "twinkle-in-the-eye" stage, when a woman
is actively trying to conceive. As an extra precaution, a
mother who has previously given birth to a baby with a
nervous-system abnormality should take a larger dose of
folic acid—5 mg daily—as soon as she is contemplating
another pregnancy. And because surprise pregnancies
can happen even to women who practice birth control,
some researchers recommend folic-acid supplementation
for all women of childbearing age, whether or not they
"plan" to become pregnant

↞ Fortification of foods. In 1996 the U.S. Food and Drug
Administration required that folic acid be added to most
prepackaged bread, flour, cornmeal, rice, noodles, and
macaroni, largely for the sake of mothers and their babies

↞ Folic-acid supplementation (in the form of a syrup) for
premature infants

THE BODY'S NEEDS

The body uses 100–200 mcg (micrograms) of folate every day,
more in people who are pregnant or ill. A normal Western diet
provides 500–700 mcg daily, but only half of this is absorbed.
Even so, the body will build up a reserve of 10–15 milligrams (1
milligram equals 1,000 micrograms); this is enough to last for
three or four months under normal conditions, but it is not
enough for a pregnancy.

FOODS PROVIDING FOLATES

One of the troubles with folic acid is that it is easily destroyed by cooking or lost by soaking in water. On the plus side, the vitamin C contained in fruits and vegetables increases the absorption of folates, but it, too, is destroyed by cooking.

> Pushpa was already pregnant when she and Eddie moved to England, leaving her big, close family behind in India. She was twenty-two and acted young for her age, because of her protected upbringing. She felt shy and strange in England; no one in the area spoke her language, and she was diffident about speaking English. That is why Pushpa didn't go to the prenatal clinic, or get to know her doctor. She felt too exhausted to face the hassle and effort, and she could not have explained in English about her headaches, her tingling hands, and her tongue's feeling funny.
>
> Despite the pregnancy, her weight had stayed the same since she left India. She did not feel like eating unfamiliar foods, so in the end she ate very little besides rice and some milk, which she thought would nourish the baby. (Cow's milk is a poor supplier of folates, and she took in hardly any vitamin C, which would have helped.)
>
> Pushpa's mother-in-law was honest and forthright. When she visited her son and daughter-in-law and observed Pushpa's condition, she took matters in hand immediately and energetically. Pushpa was marched off to the doctor's office, where her mother-in-law explained her symptoms for her. Lab tests showed that Pushpa had macrocytic anemia of pregnancy because she was short of folic acid. (Macrocytic means big cells; Pushpa's red blood cells were enlarged.) Apart from the extra demands placed on her folate reserves by the fetus, Pushpa's diet had been sadly lacking in vitamins. She was soon urged into eating what Eddie's mother called "proper dinners" consisting of meat and two vegetables. She also took folate tablets every day. Even so, little Shireen came ten days early.

Now, eight months later, the baby is thriving, Eddie is a proud father, and Pushpa is feeling well and much more confident.

Excellent Sources

Given in micrograms of folic acid per 100 grams of food substance (100 grams equals approximately 3.5 ounces).

liver	300 mcg/100 g
raw oysters	250
uncooked spinach	80
uncooked broccoli	30
uncooked cabbage	20
lettuce	20 (it takes a lot of salad greens to make 100 g)
white fish	50

Fair Sources

whole-grain bread	20 mcg/100 g
white flour	14
rice (uncooked weight)	10
bananas	10
beef	10
ham	8
eggs	8

Poor Sources

chicken, lamb, pork	3 mcg/100 g
fruits	2–5
cow's milk	0.2
human milk	0.3 (enough for a new baby)

Contains No Folic Acid

goat's milk

APLASTIC ANEMIA

Fortunately rare, aplastic anemia is a very serious form of anemia. It can affect people of any age, but the peak age of its victims is around thirty. Like many other forms of anemia, it comes
on insidiously. It involves a progressive decrease in the production of all the elements of blood: red cells, white cells, and
platelets. Because of the lack of platelets (responsible for clotting), spontaneous bleeding is likely, with nosebleeds, blood in
the urine, and little spots of bleeding in the skin, lips, and
mouth. Bruises crop up anywhere. The sufferer is vulnerable to
infections because the body's defenses, in the form of white
blood cells, are drastically reduced.

CAUSES OF APLASTIC ANEMIA

In half the cases of aplastic anemia the cause is never discovered;
these are called *idiopathic* illnesses, meaning they arise sponta-
neously, or from obscure or unknown, perhaps internal, sources.
Some known causes of aplastic anemia are listed below:

+ congenital abnormality, meaning a disorder in the genes

+ hypersensitivity (that is, an unexpected reaction) to
  certain drugs that are perfectly harmless to other
  people. Examples of drugs that trigger such a reaction
  include phenylbutazone (Butazolidin), sulfonamides,
  and gold preparations

+ the aftermath of viral hepatitis and certain other
  illnesses caused by viruses

+ toxins, including insecticides, benzene compounds
  (such as gasoline), and others

+ radiation

None of these "causes" operates by itself, since most people don't react to them by succumbing to aplastic anemia. We do not know why the manufacture of blood in the bone marrow switches off in the unlucky victims of this rare disorder.

TREATMENT AND OUTLOOK

Immunosuppressive therapy with antithymocyte globulin (ATG), antilymphocyte globulin (ALG), and/or cyclosporine is the established therapy of choice for aplastic anemia. This course of treatment has a 70 to 80 percent success rate. A bone-marrow transplant from someone whose marrow is compatible with that of the ill person, usually a relative, also gives a good chance of recovery for those under fifty. It is successful in about 80 percent of patients whose donor is a tissue-type-identical sibling. It is especially likely to be effective in children.

Other treatments include transfusions of red blood cells and platelets (the fluid part of the blood is unaffected by the disease), antibiotics to keep infections at bay, and certain steroids to stimulate the bone marrow.

There is no denying that aplastic anemia is a very dangerous illness, but the chances of improvement and recovery, if small, are real, and they make it worthwhile to continue with energetic treatment indefinitely.

Mandy was four-and-a-half and due to start school in September. She was the youngest of three, and she seemed to pick up all the viruses the others brought home from school. In the last few months she had been feeling "under the weather" more often than not. All her liveliness had been siphoned off with the last bout of sickness, and instead of improving she was getting worse. She was coughing and sniffling nonstop and looked like a little ghost. Then the frightening nosebleeds began, and little hemorrhages appeared on her lips and in her mouth. She was admitted to the children's hospital, where aplastic anemia was confirmed by blood tests.

Blood transfusions kept Mandy going for a short while, but it soon became clear that she was fighting a losing battle. Only a marrow transplant held out any hope. Her mother's bone marrow turned out to be compatible, but there were many weeks of anxiety after the operation. Would the transplant be rejected?

Mandy hovered on the brink for what seemed a lifetime, but she did survive. Now it seems hard to believe that the nightmare of three years ago even happened. Mandy is a normal seven-year-old. She was one of the lucky ones.

Chapter

8

Babies and Toddlers

There are points during our journey through life that are like the stations where we change trains. Birth is the starting point. From there, the main junctions are puberty, when we switch from childhood to the "main line," pregnancy if a woman takes that route, and then menopause, the last major upheaval in a woman's mind and body before the senior years, which finally run gently into the terminus.

Each of these life stages involves alterations in the body's functioning to accommodate a different set of priorities. The first stages concentrate on growth, and the last on running efficiently and economically. Whatever the new requirements may be, at each change new demands are placed on the blood supply, and a dip into anemia is a common risk at these times.

It is easy to understand how newborn babies, growing at a phenomenal rate on a very limited diet of milk, can run short of the ingredients for making blood after age four or five months. The situation is somewhat similar during the growth spurt of puberty, which, for girls, includes the major event of menarche, the start of monthly bleeding from the womb. This phenomenon is controlled by the sex hormones, particularly estrogen, but it may take several months before the arrangements work smoothly. Meanwhile, girls may experience an excessive loss of blood during the early menstrual periods, especially those occurring before the regular release of egg cells. Losing blood leads directly to anemia.

At the other end of the reproductive phase, menopause, the process is repeated in reverse. Hormonal control may falter at this stage, too, again producing irregular periods, some of them heavy and prone to what is graphically called "flooding." The average loss of blood per period is 30 milliliters (about 1 fluid ounce), but it may be as much as 175 milliliters. Pregnancy also places a drain on a woman's resources since it involves building and nourishing a brand-new individual from her own body and blood. Finally, senior citizens, who often have a restricted diet, present another risk group for anemia.

The good news is that anemia in any life stage can be prevented and, if worse comes to worst, treated. For prevention, a balanced, well-constructed diet is essential during all life changes, one that includes vitamins, minerals (especially iron), and plenty of energy from among the three basic macronutrients: carbohydrate, protein, and fat. Also essential is tuning in and paying attention to your body, with a vigilant eye trained on catching any of the early signs and symptoms of anemia. To help you achieve these goals no matter where you are in life, the next five chapters deal with the risks for and prevention of anemia in the various life stages.

BOTTLE OR BREAST?

A baby's first year of life is also the first risk period for anemia—he is growing so fast that he is rapidly using up his iron reserves and cannot replace them fast enough. For his first four months his diet is, and should be, exclusively milk. It may be breast milk or formula, but neither contains adequate supplies of iron, so he is operating on the iron stores he started with fresh from the uterus.

Breast-feeding is a unique experience that only women can enjoy, and a gift that only a mother can give to her baby. All the health authorities agree that breast milk is the best all around for a baby. The "pluses" of breast-feeding and breast milk include:

+ no danger of contamination

+ contains a range of anti-infective agents, from immuno-globulins to interferon

+ reduces the risk of stomach and gut (gastrointestinal) upsets, as well as other infections, such as bronchitis, meningitis, otitis (ear infection), and cystitis (bladder infection)

+ reduces the risk of allergies and diabetes

+ the temperature is perfect

+ baby must work harder to release breast milk, and the flow is variable. Thus, sucking from a breast develops his jaw, so his teeth are less likely to be crowded

+ iron, which is in short supply in all types of milk, is better absorbed from breast milk than from cow's milk or formula—an anti-anemia feature

+ deepens and enriches the bond between mother and child

Reasons Not to Breast-Feed

Breast-feeding may get good press, but a mother should not feel pressured to do it. Perhaps the circumstances are not right—lack of privacy, work commitments, such problems as inverted nipples, or simply her feelings. If you really do not want to breast-feed—DON'T. A happy mother is far more important to a baby than even the most wonderful milk.

A mother needs to feel fit and to have been eating properly—both during the pregnancy and after—to take on the job of feeding her baby from her own resources. Breast-feeding is a definite no-no if a mother has either of two conditions: HIV or tuberculosis. Additionally, certain drugs and medicines come through in the milk and may harm the baby: diazepam (Valium), reserpine, morphine derivatives, indomethacin, lithium, cannabis, and other less commonplace recreational drugs. Radioactive and other anticancer drugs are unsuitable for a nursing mother. She should also avoid close contact with insecticides and dry-cleaning solvent.

Formula Feeding

Breast may be best if the mother encounters no problems and feels happy and comfortable with it. For mothers who decide against breast-feeding, for whatever combination of reasons, modern formula is so cunningly modified that it closely resembles breast milk, except it includes more iron. Don't feel your baby is deprived if she is fed formula instead of breast milk—so long as you spend time loving and cuddling her. (Untreated cow's milk has a different composition from human milk, since it is laying the foundations for a very different animal, so it is unsuitable for a baby.)

GUIDELINES FOR BREAST-FEEDING

Leila was the sort of person who read the small print on labels, so she wanted to know exactly what she should do about the everyday drugs, such as coffee and tobacco, while she was nursing baby Chris. Here's what she learned:

Cigarettes: Smoking while nursing substantially reduces the output of a mother's milk. Additionally, growing up in a household with smokers increases the risk to a young baby of developing sniffles, colds, asthma, and chest infections. Leila decided to give up smoking altogether—at any rate for a few months, by which time the craving should have subsided.

Alcohol: A baby receives proportionately as much alcohol in her system as the nursing mother has in her blood. A maximum of one drink a day can do no harm, and beer may even stimulate milk production. Excessive alcohol can have dire effects on a baby, particularly on her brain development. Instead, drink to your baby's health in milk or water, both of which are useful in making milk.

Coffee and tea: As with the alcohol in alcoholic drinks, a nursing baby takes in any caffeine circulating through her mother's system. Enjoying a few cups of coffee or tea will do no harm—if drunk one at a time, well spaced throughout the day—but too much will keep your baby awake in the night, something you definitely want to avoid!

What You Eat Can Affect Your Milk

Diet does not influence the amounts of the basic food ingredients—protein, lactose (milk sugar), fat, and calcium—in a mother's milk, but it can affect levels of several of the B-complex vitamins (B-1, B-2, B-12, folic acid), as well as vitamins C and D, and iron. Iron, vitamin B-12, and folate are needed in the nursing mother's diet—probably in large amounts provided only by supplements—to ward off the different anemias related to deficiencies in those substances.

Just as important as *what* you eat is *how much*. Nursing mothers need five hundred to seven hundred additional calories per day.

Gemma had intended to bottle-feed and go back to her prestigious job in merchant banking as soon as her baby was a month old. However, little Angela was so sweet and funny that Gemma decided she needed a full three months off to give her a good start and to get to know her better.

Gemma had always been figure conscious, and now she was eager to have a flat tummy again ASAP. Originally she had planned to bottle-feed Angela, but then she read that the

---

In addition to her increased caloric requirements, the extra nutrients a nursing mother needs to eat daily over and above her normal diet are:

Water: 1.5 pints

Protein: 11 grams

Calcium: 550 milligrams (contained in 1 pint of milk or
    2 cartons of yogurt)

Vitamin C: 30 mg

Folate: 60 mg

Vitamin D: 10 micrograms (strict vegetarians especially need
    to be careful to get enough vitamin D during pregnancy)

French—always in the forefront of fashion—insisted that their models breast-feed. It helped tighten up the abdominal muscles, and the breasts regained their pre-pregnancy contour better after six weeks of breast-feeding. So Gemma breast-fed her baby, and found it unexpectedly soothing.

Her gynecologist approved of this, but firmly discouraged Gemma against her plan to start a slimming diet immediately, "to give Nature a helping hand." She told Gemma that attempts at weight reduction in the middle of breast-feeding could upset her fat metabolism and possibly produce toxic substances, such as ketones, that could affect her and the baby.

Susie was a natural at breast-feeding, and at motherhood in general. Little Avril was a happy, contented baby who got the hang of sucking from the start and slept through most of the nights. She and her mother both enjoyed the feeding times, and Susie continued with breast-feeding for nearly five months. When she stopped, she continued eating the slightly increased food intake she had been advised to take while nursing.

It only takes a few too many calories on a regular basis to add pounds. Susie was not worried—she was enchanted with Avril. But her husband was unhappy to see his pretty young wife lumbering around like an elephant, and he was not as wrapped up in the baby as Susie was. When Avril could throw a ball it would be a different matter. The concerted efforts of the women who cared about Susie—her mother, sister, friends, and coworkers—finally convinced her to pay attention to her health, start exercising, and trim her diet.

WEANING

Once your baby reaches the age of about four months, neither your wonderful breast milk nor the best scientifically constructed formula is enough to nourish her. In particular, she will be running out of the iron and zinc stored in her body, which increases her chances of having problems with iron-deficiency anemia. The first indications of anemia in a baby are that the baby becomes quieter and moves less.

In some cases, especially with a vegan or vegetarian breast-feeding mother, it is vitamin B-12 that is inadequate in the diet and therefore the less common B-12–deficiency anemia that threatens. Folic-acid deficiency is another possible cause of anemia in a breast-fed baby, unless the mother has been taking folate supplements, as is usual in the United States.

Baby's Dietary Calendar

0–4 months Milk only (water if thirsty)

4–6 months Add cereals in milk

6–7 months Pureed vegetables; mashed banana

8–9 months Finger foods—melba toast, bananas, chopped cooked vegetables, e.g., carrots. Commercial preparations can be introduced

9 months Meat, sieved or canned; orange juice from a cup; pureed fruit; mashed potato; porridge

10 months Egg yolk; bite-sized chunks of family food

12 months Whole egg; cheese; bread; and most foods that you eat

The usual signal from a baby that she is ready to move on from a purely milk diet is her still being hungry at the end of a feeding. Baby's first "solid" food is a cereal mixed to a runny consistency with milk—either formula made up according to the package directions or expressed breast milk. Most women use formula for this purpose. Rice is less likely than wheat to cause sensitivity, so it is normally the first cereal introduced. It is usually fortified with iron, which the baby needs urgently starting at the age of four to five months. She also needs vitamin C, which helps with the absorption of iron as well as providing other benefits; from the age of nine months she will be able to get this in a citrus drink, although some mothers try to introduce juice earlier by diluting it.

In addition, the following points are important to remember:

↞ Babies under age four months cannot swallow solids and cannot digest starches or fats; they don't yet have the necessary digestive enzymes.

↞ Attempts at feeding from a spoon before age four months are likely to set off a reflex of rejecting it.

↞ Sieved or pureed spinach, turnip, or beet given before age four to six months may turn hemoglobin into methemoglobin, which is useless. This increases the risk of anemia.

↞ Unboiled cow's milk given in the first six months may cause bleeding in the stomach, which can also lead to anemia.

↞ Eggs given in the first six months can cause allergy.

↞ The most critical nutrients after age four months are protein and iron.

FUSSY FEEDERS

Jessica, like any child, was thrilled by mirrors. Catching sight of her own reflection, she gave it a brilliant smile. She was exactly the same age as Jonathan, the young scientist visiting at her house that day. He was examining a small object, holding it first in one hand then the other, feeling it for texture and testing it for taste. They were celebrating their first birthday; their mothers, Kate and Lindy, had met in the maternity ward a year ago. Both moms were in despair. Until now, both babies had taken their food by spoon or cup without any trouble, but in the last week or so they had been refusing even their favorite foods—and they were hardly putting on any weight. Kate and Lindy were reassured when they saw the doctor and she explained.

A lot of toddlers between the ages of one and three go through a period of poor eating—with a special dislike for vegetables—and worrying their mothers in the process. One big reason for this is that babies do not continue growing at such breakneck speed when they reach age one, neither in weight nor height. Their appetite slows down to match.

The other important reason is that these little children are busy discovering their independence and practicing making their own choices. They soon find out about the attractive taste of chocolate cake and ice cream, and may try to insist that these make up most of their diet. It is a phase that passes, so long as parents continue serving the ordinary healthy foods before the treats. To ward off infections and anemia a toddler still needs protein, vegetables, and the foods containing iron and vitamins. It often works to give him or her four or five small meals throughout the day, rather than three dauntingly large ones—but pressuring them is counterproductive, as Kate and Lindy discovered. After learning from their pediatrician that they needn't worry, both moms relaxed a little, but continued to offer their youngsters a balanced diet—and Jessica and Jonathan continued to thrive.

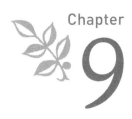

Chapter

9

Preadolescent and Adolescent Girls

Preadolescence and adolescence, the next periods in a young woman's life for reassessment and readjustment of her risk factors for anemia, mean total physical and psychological chaos. Shakespeare, in *The Winter's Tale*, put his finger on it: "I would rather there were no age between ten and three-and-twenty, or that youth would sleep out the rest...." The years of transition from childhood to womanhood are the most difficult and exciting of one's life. They involve more rapid bodily growth than at any time since babyhood, plus brand-new, revolutionary emotional and intellectual development.

For example, between ages ten and twenty, the muscle weight of an average girl increases from about ten to twenty pounds. The uterus, which is mostly muscle, gets much bigger. Muscle is mainly made of protein. Protein is also needed to make red blood cells, so to avoid anemia the diet must include a plentiful supply of it. The amount of calcium stored in the body, mostly in the rapidly growing bones, increases from 300 to 750 grams (from about 10 to about 24 ounces) during adolescence, calling for a generous intake of dairy products.

But the body needs more than just meat and milk. For allover growth, the body requires optimum supplies of all the other nutrients, obtained by eating a wide variety of good foods. The ideal diet during adolescence includes enough fruits, vegetables, and whole grains to make up 50 to 55 percent of total caloric intake, with plenty of protein (making up 15 to 20 percent of calories), a small amount of fat to complete the balance (25 to 35 percent of calories), and adequate fiber (which adds no calories to the diet).

Exercise is another component of a healthy lifestyle during the teen years. It is necessary in order to rev up the circulation, which in turn increases efficiency in carrying the vital nutrients to every part of the body. Exercise also keeps the bones and muscles in first-class working order.

LIFESTYLE RISK FACTORS IN ADOLESCENCE

Poor Diet and Exercise Habits

Unfortunately, what often happens in adolescence is the exact opposite of what the body needs. Teenagers, especially boys, are notorious for their huge appetites—at times downing four thousand calories a day, largely from sweets and fatty foods. And while girls may tend to follow a diet closer to the ideal than boys, truth be told, many youngsters of both sexes have terrible eating habits. For the first time in their lives they are taking responsibility for their own food intake. Their meals are often irregular and based on junk food—palatable and easy to eat, but fatty and scant in vitamins, iron, and often protein. They frequently miss a meal, usually breakfast, which can account for poor classroom performance. Choosing for themselves means they tend to go for "treat foods": those that are easily available, are conveniently placed next to the supermarket checkouts, and require no preparation. Such convenience foods are usually full of empty calories and are useless for building or repairing tissues or making blood. They include foods high in sugar and fats, plus diet soft drinks—which do not even offer calories for energy. Alcohol enters a girl's social life around this time and brings with it a bundle of dangers, including teen pregnancy. Accidents related to alcohol are a major cause of death for both sexes in the fifteen- to twenty-four-year age group.

What can a concerned parent do to encourage healthy eating during these independent years? If you can't monitor every bite your teenager puts in her mouth when she's out of your sight, at least you can control what's available when she's under your roof. Teenagers are habitual snackers, especially after school. Left entirely up to their own devices, they tend to gravitate toward chocolate bars, cookies, chips, and fries—foods containing neither iron nor vitamins. However, with a little planning, you can influence the choices available when your teenager is at home. It is vital to make sure that a variety of fruits, unsalted nuts, and vegetables such as carrots and celery is always on hand. Milk drinks, cheese, whole-wheat crackers, and fresh and dried fruits are "good" snacks, providing calcium, protein, vitamin B-12, vitamin C, and fiber.

Only too frequently, a couch-potato diet goes hand in hand with a couch-potato lifestyle. At this age girls more often than boys may give up exercise altogether, starting with team sports. They may never regain the exercise habit or take an interest in sports, except for watching their favorite sports heroes on TV. Mothers, especially, but also fathers can help to inspire their daughters by exercising regularly themselves—but if a parent's own exercise program isn't what they think it "should" be, it is not worth getting a guilt complex over.

Eating Disorders

As if faulty eating habits and too little exercise weren't bad enough, even more likely to lead to anemia are the two main eating disorders, which affect girls and young women almost exclusively: anorexia nervosa and bulimia nervosa. In anorexia ner-

Calculating Body Mass Index (BMI)

Step 1. Convert pounds to kilograms: Weight of 120 pounds divided by 2.2 equals 54.5 kg

Step 2. Convert inches to meters: Height of 65 inches divided by 39.37 equals 1.65 meters

Step 3. Square the meters: 1.65 times 1.65 equals 2.72

Step 4. Calculate BMI: 54.5 (weight in kg) divided by 2.72 (height in meters, squared) equals BMI of 20.04

---

vosa the victim deliberately starves herself and often exercises excessively; in bulimia she eats the food, often in "binge" episodes, but later purges it from her body by vomiting or use of laxatives. In either condition the body is deprived of the ingredients necessary to make blood, especially protein and minerals.

Signs that may indicate bulimia include a tendency to leave the table immediately after a meal, in order to vomit in secrecy. Repeated vomiting can lead to swelling of the salivary glands, which shows up as soft bumps at the base of the ears or just under the chin. If the behavior continues for many years the swellings become hard and permanent. Also, the salivary glands often become infected, hard, and painful. Other behaviors potentially indicative of bulimia include binge eating, awareness of abnormal eating patterns (unlike anorexics, who see nothing "wrong" with their behavior), a fear of being unable to stop eating, attempts to eat inconspicuously, depressed mood following an eating binge, abdominal pain, frequent weight fluctuations, suicidal thoughts, frequent use of laxatives or diuretics, excessive sleeping, loneliness, and anger.

Spotting anorexia is somewhat simpler. If the weight of a five-foot-three-inch adolescent girl falls below ninety-five pounds, it is a warning that she is teetering on the dangerous borders of anorexia. Another way of gauging a healthy body size is by body mass index (BMI), calculated by dividing weight in kilograms by height in meters squared. A BMI of eighteen or less spells anorexia. (See the table below for an example of calculating BMI, including converting pounds and inches to kilograms and meters.)

ANEMIA IN TEENAGE GIRLS

Anemia—low-quality blood—is, unfortunately, common among adolescent girls. Over the long term, an unhealthy lifestyle, especially an inadequate diet, can bring on the disease's signs and symptoms gradually. Another cause of anemia at this age is loss of blood, which, by contrast, produces anemia quickly.

A major blood loss, as from a serious accident, produces instant anemia, calling for a blood transfusion. A less dramatic loss of blood, but enough to cause anemia, often occurs in teenage girls. This is the menorrhagia—or excessive menstrual bleeding—of puberty (*meno-* has to do with the menstrual cycle; *-rrhagia* means *bursting forth*). It can crop up during the early monthly cycles after menarche (the first bleed) has occurred, but before ovulation (egg production) has gotten under way. The bleeding may be regular but excessive, or it may be continuous. Three or four months on a contraceptive pill will control the situation, but both types of bleeding will settle down once ovulation has become established.

Effects of Anemia on This Age Group

Listed below are the symptoms that may indicate anemia in an adolescent girl:

+ Poor concentration, making for difficulties with studying—a disaster during the school years

+ Looking pale. Pale skin by itself is of no concern—unless it is accompanied by one or more of the other symptoms

+ Lack of energy. It feels different from common adolescent lethargy, which is more a matter of mood

* Picky appetite, unlike the normal adolescent situation of eating enormously (boys) or periodically going on weight-reduction diets (girls). Naturally finicky eaters usually outgrow this pattern by adolescence

* Occasional insomnia—a rarity in a teenager

* Cold hands and feet, sometimes including dead-white fingers even in warm weather

* Feeling dizzy and sometimes fainting

* Uncomfortable awareness of heartbeat (palpitations)

The different types of anemia can all lead to these symptoms, plus others, depending on the type and severity of the anemia. For more detail about the specific symptoms and signs of the various types of anemia, see Chapters 3 through 7.

What to Do

All cases of anemia in adolescence call for a complete overhaul of the adolescent's lifestyle and diet, with an emphasis on increasing consumption of iron-containing foods such as red meat, dark chocolate, oatmeal, bran cereal, sardines, and legumes; enough animal products to boost the stores of vitamin B-12, including meat, fish, eggs, milk, and cheese; and, for folic acid, green leafy vegetables.

More drastic treatment may also be needed. Depending on the type and severity of anemia, such therapy might include a blood transfusion (in the case of sudden, serious blood loss), supplementation in the form of pills with iron or folic acid (see Chapters 4 and 7 respectively for more about these anemias), or injections of vitamin B-12 (see Chapters 5 and 6). Treating the serious but very rare condition of aplastic anemia may entail a regimen of drugs to suppress the autoimmune system or even a bone-marrow transplant (see Chapter 7).

Alison was fourteen when she began developing ideals and enthusiasms. She supported all the wildlife projects—Save the Badgers, the Elephants, the Whales, and the Hedgehogs. Naturally enough, she could not bear the thought of eating meat. From being a moderate vegetarian she gradually became practically vegan.

She had been on this strict diet for over two years when she began having symptoms. First, she often noticed the feeling of pins and needles in her hands. This was awkward when she wanted to play the piano, especially since added to that she found she kept forgetting the notes. A nagging backache did not help, and she felt permanently tired.

Alison had slipped into the type of anemia caused by lack of vitamin B-12, a nutrient that is found in reliable amounts only in foods from animal sources—milk, eggs, meat, cheese, and fish. No combination of vegetables can substitute for these. The best known early-warning symptoms of a person's supply of B-12 running out include a sore, red tongue and cracks at the corners of the mouth. These did not upset Alison as much as the symptoms that indicated problems in her nervous system—the pins and needles, forgetfulness, and loss of ability to concentrate on her music. For years she had cherished secret dreams of becoming a concert pianist, and her enthusiasm for music matched what she felt about wildlife.

In the end Alison was persuaded to compromise and eat some foods containing vitamin B-12. She started with milk, then added an occasional egg, and finally a sliver of meat now and then—all obtained according to the standards of compassionate farming. While the effect of her improved nourishment was building up, Alison had a few B-12 injections to give her B-12 status a rapid boost.

10

Pregnant Women

The ideal time for a girl to start preparing to give her kids a head start in life is during her own childhood! Nothing boosts the chances of having a healthy, strong body in adulthood like building the foundation of good health and dietary habits beginning in childhood. Ideally, each child's parents should see to it that she gets plenty of protein, iron, and vitamins, plus the energy foods: carbohydrates and fats. Calcium from dairy products builds strong bones in a girl, and exercise—school sports, swimming, walking, running, and social games such as tennis—help to develop muscles and check any tendency to get flabby. Strong bones and muscles are exactly what a woman needs years later to give birth.

Not all children, of course, have equal access to good nutrition. Fortunately, there are many ways a young woman can increase the possibility of having a successful, healthy pregnancy once she reaches the age when she's responsible for taking care of herself. The first tool she can take advantage of is awareness—of the consequences of her sexual behavior, and of how her lifestyle affects her health.

Specifically preparing for the possibility of becoming a mother starts when a young woman begins having sex. She needs to be aware that pregnancy can occur as something a woman has been hoping for, as a lovely surprise, as something of an inconvenience just now—or as a ghastly shock. Even a woman who practices birth control can get pregnant. If she's using the contraceptive Pill, for example, she might forget to take it on occasion, or she might have a bout of diarrhea that washes it out of her system at the crucial time. Because anything can happen, women of childbearing age who are sexually active would be wise to take care of themselves and their bodies with an eye to any future offspring they might conceive.

Gemma was not a model, but she liked to think she had the figure for it. At twenty-one she looked smashing, and, if anything, even better at thirty-one. Her looks plus her experience were moving her up the career ladder in a gratifying manner. Bob, her boyfriend, was ten years older, which meant he was comfortably established, with a nice apartment in the city, a cottage on the coast, and a car for each of them.

When Gemma was thirty-eight (she could easily have passed for twenty-five), she decided to put her job on hold, have a baby, and get back to work a month later. It did not work out so easily. Bob, who had been an athlete in his twenties and thirties, was now—to be truthful—soft and paunchy, with a taste for French wines and a liking for stick-to-the-ribs meals suitable for a lumberjack. Gemma persisted with her vegetarian, weight-restricting diet on the grounds that it was healthy. Certainly it was full of antioxidants and fiber from all the fruits and vegetables.

After two years of trying to get pregnant by having sex more often—especially around the middle of her menstrual cycle, when she was ovulating—Gemma finally conceived. Her heart was set on having this baby, so she was scared when the obstetrician told her she was anemic. It was essential for her to follow the dietary rules he gave her, plus boost her iron stores by taking supplements.

FOOD AND DIET IN PREGNANCY: INCREASED DEMANDS

Additional nutrients are needed during pregnancy, especially starting in the twentieth week, but the actual quantity of food—that is, the intake of calories—for most well-fed Western women hardly needs to increase at all from normal. Specifically, nourishment is needed for:

✦ Building tissue in the mother's body, especially for development of the breasts and womb, and of the baby-feeding factory, the placenta. A woman will also put on three to four pounds of fat during pregnancy, mainly deposited over the hips and thighs. You can imagine how cross Gemma was about this, but most new mothers are able to shed the unwanted fat after the baby is born. Breast-feeding helps, since the extra store of bodily fat is intended especially to provide for the milk supply

✦ Maintenance work on the mother's body, specifically to prevent anemia from the increased demands on her blood supply, and to replace the calcium "borrowed" from her teeth and bones by the fetus

✦ Making a whole new person: the fetus that becomes a baby. This means building bone, blood, muscle, brain and nerves, and myriad other tissues

✦ The sixty thousand extra calories demanded by pregnancy. However, a woman needn't eat all that extra food. She naturally tends to get less exercise during pregnancy, her metabolism is particularly efficient, and some calories are saved from her not having periods

Although there is no need in most cases to increase caloric intake in general, half a dozen critical ingredients in the diet *do* need to increase. These are the following:

Protein: 70 grams daily, an increase of 10 g

Folic acid: 600 micrograms daily, an increase of 200 mcg

Calcium: 1,200 milligrams daily, an increase of 200 mg

Iron: 30 milligrams daily, an increase of 12 mg

Zinc: 15 milligrams daily, an increase of 3 mg

Iodine: 175 micrograms daily, an increase of 25 mcg

(Note the large increases in required amounts of folic acid and iron, two of the anti-anemia nutrients.)

In the United States, obstetricians routinely prescribe prenatal (meaning *before birth*) vitamin and mineral supplements to pregnant women to ensure that they get the increased levels they need of these and other nutrients.

Folic Acid (Folate)

Folic acid, one of the B vitamins, is the most important nutrient for making DNA, the blueprint for a baby's individual development, which is replicated over and over throughout a person's life. Disastrous problems in a baby's nervous system, for instance spina bifida, can be prevented by a sufficient intake of folate, especially around six weeks into the pregnancy—that is, two weeks after the menstrual period is first missed. In fact, folate levels should stay topped up from the moment a woman thinks she has conceived, and it is impossible to know for sure when this has happened. That is why the U.S. Food and Nutrition Board recommends a relatively high level of folic acid intake for even nonpregnant women of childbearing age (400 mcg daily). Women also need adequate levels of dietary folate to reduce the risk of anemia.

Sources of Folic Acid

Very good: bran, endive, yeast extract

Good: broccoli (not the stalk), spinach, Brussels sprouts, nuts, kidneys, peas, bran cereal

Fair: avocado, oatmeal, beets, egg yolk, whole-grain bread, peanut butter, oranges

Negligible: legumes (the pea and bean family; note that they lose 80 percent of their folate content during cooking)

Liver provides an excellent supply of folate, but eating a lot of liver carries the risk of delivering an excess of vitamin A, which can cause abnormalities in the baby's development.

Folate supplements, in particular, are usually given routinely during pregnancy.

Iron

Obtaining sufficient dietary iron during pregnancy is an absolute must. But, apparently, many women fail to do so. The World Health Organization in 1992 estimated that 17 percent of pregnant women in the United States suffer from iron-deficiency anemia, a condition that can affect the health of both mother and baby. The fetus requires 300 mg of iron, the placenta 50 mg, and the blood lost during labor means another 200 mg of iron that will need replacing, amounting to a total of about 550 mg. All this iron must be obtained from the mother's diet.

There is also an increased amount of blood in circulation, particularly after the twelfth week of pregnancy, corresponding to another 500 mg of iron, but this is normally supplied by internal borrowing from the iron stores in the mother's body. It is necessary for a woman to keep her iron reserves well supplied if she is contemplating pregnancy.

Hemoglobin is the vital red pigment of the blood needed for transporting oxygen to all parts of the body, and iron is necessary for the production of hemoglobin. The level of hemoglobin in the blood is reduced by about 10 percent in pregnancy, and so is the concentration of iron in the serum. These losses can be modified but not completely prevented by taking extra iron. The doctor's rule of thumb is to prescribe iron supplements if a woman's hemoglobin slips below 11 g/dl (grams per deciliter) and if her red blood cells include some that are noticeably small.

Iron supplements usually come in the form of tablets. The problem is that they often cause constipation, already likely to be troublesome in pregnancy. Other common side effects include indigestion and loose stools. Liquid preparations are an alternative, less likely to cause indigestion, while injections are another possibility for anyone unable to tolerate the tablets.

Sources of Iron

Some foods, such as meat, contain a concentrated supply of iron, while others, like watercress, require a huge amount to provide a little iron. This is one reason why vegetarians may run short of

Iron Content of Some Foods (mg per 100 g of food substance)	
Beef	3.5 mg/100 g
Lamb	2.7
Oatmeal	3.8
Cooked legumes, e.g., baked beans, tofu	1.4–3.5
Boiled egg	1.9
Dark chocolate	2.4
AllBran cereal	20
Blackstrap molasses	9
Bread, white or whole-grain	1.6–2.7
Watercress and other green leafy vegetables	0.7–2.2
Milk, all types	0.05 (very little)

iron—they cannot eat enough spinach! The best-absorbed provider of iron is red meat, especially lean beef—as well as blood sausage, if you can stomach it. Liver contains plenty of iron, but it carries the risk of delivering an excess of vitamin A.

Calcium

Calcium is needed for the baby's framework of bones and his budding teeth. Since calcium for the baby is taken from the mother's own calcium supplies, if she's not getting enough of the mineral in her diet, the calcium in her bones and teeth could be depleted. Fortunately, Nature lends a helping hand and enables Mom to absorb calcium more efficiently than usual.

Extra dietary calcium is easily available in milk and cheese. Half a liter of milk (just over three-quarters of a pint) or two ounces of Cheddar cheese provide 600 mg of calcium—about half the normal daily requirement.

Zinc

The mineral zinc functions in the body as part of about three hundred different enzymes. Like iron, zinc tends to run short during pregnancy; its blood level drops by 30 percent in pregnant women. Supplementing with zinc does not affect the level of the mineral in the body during pregnancy, but good dietary sources are oysters (the best), red meat, organ meat, shellfish, whole grains, nuts, and cheese. Soy products reduce its absorption.

Protein

Protein is a major building material and one of the foods metabolized more rapidly and efficiently in pregnancy. A woman will find that this faster burn provides her with personal central heating—a boon in the winter, when everyone else is shivering. There is no need for her to eat much more protein during pregnancy than she would normally—unless she is a vegetarian. Proteins are found in meat, fish, cheese, milk, and eggs, all from animal sources, and in the form of vegetable protein from peas and beans, nuts, and, most prominently, soy. Of the vegetable proteins, only soy provides all the essential amino acids, the building blocks for human protein (such as muscle). However, no plant sources supply vitamin B-12, which is necessary to avoid B-12-deficiency anemia, including pernicious anemia, and some disorders of the nervous system.

Vegetarians such as Gemma risk depriving their fetuses of the protein they need. The stricter the diet the greater the risk to development, affecting the baby's brain in particular. Pregnant women especially must not make such a decision lightly. They need to educate themselves about the risks inherent in a meatless diet and about the rigorous dietary requirements vegetarians must follow to get all the protein they and their baby need. Vegan mothers certainly cannot provide all their babies require from their own diet, either during pregnancy or if they attempt breast-feeding. They must supplement with B-12 and iron, and certainly must make sure they get several servings each day of *complete* protein—such as that contained in soy—for the fetus to thrive. Even lacto-ovovegetarians, those who eat milk and eggs, must take supplements of vitamin B-12 and iron during pregnancy. Eating nuts and legumes helps, but the fetus will stand the best chance for good health if its mother eats red meat—not in large quantities but regularly.

WEIGHT GAIN

Over the course of a pregnancy a woman will put on between 15 and 50 pounds; most should aim for an increase of around 26 pounds. This works out to a gain of a quarter pound per week for the first ten weeks, increasing to two-thirds of a pound weekly for the remaining forty weeks.

A woman who smokes during pregnancy will gain less weight, and her baby is more likely to be underweight at birth, increasing the infant's vulnerability to sickness. Becoming overweight during pregnancy also involves risks to both mother and baby. The mother is more likely to develop gestational diabetes (pregnancy-related diabetes) or toxemia (pregnancy-related high blood pressure). A high-salt or low-salt diet does not affect this type of high blood pressure—nor does any other item in the diet—but a shortage of calcium may make matters worse.

> Judy was twenty-four when she became pregnant. She had always had a weight problem; at five feet three inches she weighed 154 pounds. (Her ideal weight would have been 112 pounds.) The obstetrician explained that 6 to 8 pounds of the usual 26-pound weight gain in pregnancy is fat, and that therefore Judy should aim to put on only 14 to 16 pounds total.
>
> The problem was that Judy had developed a passion for sweet rolls, the kind with thick white icing on top, and controlling her appetite for these treats was difficult. What shook her was the doctor telling her that she had toxemia, and that there could be a danger of losing the baby if it became worse. This news shocked Judy into watching her diet, and she managed to keep her weight steady during the last month of pregnancy. She finished only 2 pounds heavier than her target. The birth would have been quicker and easier if Judy had been slimmer, but the baby was particularly beautiful. He clocked in at 8 pounds.

THE ANNOYANCES OF PREGNANCY

Pregnancy brings with it some common but tiresome problems, none of them dangerous.

Morning Sickness

A woman finding herself nauseated every morning is what often leads to the diagnosis of pregnancy. Morning sickness usually sweeps over a person when she first wakes up, but it can come on in the evening or any other time. Typically, she feels nauseous as soon as she lifts her head off the pillow; some women actually vomit. The trigger is probably low blood sugar, and it usually helps to nibble a couple of plain sweet cookies—shortbread or graham crackers or something similar. Oddly enough, a pregnant woman is likely to put on weight during this phase, whether she's vomiting or not.

Occasionally, a woman can develop a very severe form of morning sickness, called *hyperemesis gravidarum* (Latin for *severe sickness of pregnant women*). If that happens she should consult her doctor. If she's not careful, the complete loss of appetite that often accompanies severe morning sickness can lead to an inadequate intake of the nutrients she needs in order to prevent anemia.

Constipation

Constipation affects at least 50 percent of mothers-to-be. It is due to the relaxation of the autonomic (automatic) muscles in the abdomen, to allow for the stretching of the tissues as the fetus gets bigger. Constipation often leads to hemorrhoids from the pressure on the back and the straining. These are likely to bleed and may contribute to the development of anemia.

To help with constipation, increase your intake of wholegrain bread, bran and bran cereals, fruits, and vegetables to increase the bulk of the stools and to loosen their consistency.

Heartburn

Heartburn involves a burning sensation behind the breastbone. The upward pressure from the uterus makes heartburn more likely in pregnancy. (The same principle—upward pressure from an oversize abdomen—is responsible for a higher incidence of heartburn in obese individuals.) It is less likely to occur if a person eats four to six small meals spread throughout the day, instead of two or three substantial ones.

Cravings

Food fads, cravings, and aversions may replace a woman's usual likes and dislikes during pregnancy, for no obvious reason. The cravings are most often for sweet foods—for instance, fudge or chocolate ice cream—and in rare cases she may have a yen for nonfoods, such as chalk. There is no special way of coping with these oddities, except exercising common sense. Again, failing to get a balanced diet during this crucial time because you're filled up on sweets can lead to anemia.

What Not to Eat

Since infections from the *Listeria* and salmonella bacteria are much more serious in pregnancy, avoid eating:

- Unpasteurized milk
- Soft cheeses, such as Brie or Camembert
- Paté
- Raw or lightly cooked eggs; for example, soft-boiled or soft-scrambled
- Custard, if left in the open to cool
- Precooked foods
- Delicatessen foods
- Meat or fish pies
- Quiche

If you do eat these foods, make sure they have been heated all the way through to a temperature above 140 degrees Fahrenheit (microwaving is ideal).

Most of all, remember that the choices you make about food are the best way you can help yourself enjoy a successful, healthy pregnancy—and help yourself avoid anemia at any stage of life.

Chapter 11

Menopause

The particular significance of menopause is that it is the last major upheaval that affects a woman's mind and body, setting her course for the next three or four decades. To enjoy these years to the fullest, she needs to be fit. One disorder that can spoil this time in a woman's life is anemia, which can creep up on her silently and catch her unawares. As mentioned earlier, the menopausal shift in hormonal levels may produce irregular menstrual periods, some of them quite heavy and prone to "flooding." The resulting loss of blood is a distinct risk factor for anemia. In addition, other health situations specific to the menopausal years bring with them special considerations for preventing and treating anemia.

The mildest case of anemia reduces a person's vitality and dampens her enthusiasm. In a moderately severe case even the everyday tasks become a burden, the sufferer falls prey to any passing infection, her energy level registers at zero, her memory is like a sieve, and she cannot concentrate. Anemia also provides an unwelcome boost to the aging process. Many of these conditions are also associated with menopause, meaning they would be made worse by undetected, untreated anemia. Chances are a woman experiencing these unpleasant effects won't receive any sympathy; indeed, both she and others may write off her symptoms as menopausal changes. Therefore, she needs to remain especially vigilant for the warning signs of anemia during this "change of life." This chapter addresses each of these issues.

THE MECHANISM OF MENOPAUSE

The hallmark of being a woman, and the whole future of the human race, resides in the oocytes or egg cells. Each one of these is enclosed in a tiny sac or follicle within the ovaries, and each one is precious. Unlike men, who can continue manufacturing sperm, their small but essential contribution to making a baby, into their seventies, we females have all the egg cells we are ever going to have on the day we are born.

The follicles are more than sperm equivalents. The granulosa cells (*granulosa* means *grainy*) in the linings of the follicles act like miniature estrogen factories. Estrogen is the most important female hormone, closely bound up with control of the menstrual cycle, pregnancy, and especially with menopause and its symptoms. The granulosa cells also produce the hormone inhibin, which assists with ovulation (the release of an egg cell every month).

You would think that having two million follicles, the average starting count, would be overkill, and that a woman could never run short. But throughout the fertile years, usually from ages fifteen to forty-five, the number of follicles steadily declines. This falloff escalates dramatically around age thirty-five, or sooner if a woman's periods started early. Fewer follicles means fewer egg cells and dwindling chances of one of them being fertilized; that is why a woman's fertility decreases so dramatically in her mid- to late thirties. Twelve to fourteen years later, when the number of remaining follicles inexorably drops to twenty-five thousand, the menopausal process kicks in. Menopause officially occurs when a woman has had her very last period. However, because menstruation can be so irregular in the years leading up to menopause, sometimes it's impossible to know it has happened until a woman has stopped having periods for several months.

Heredity strongly influences when all of this will happen; a woman is likely to follow the same time frame as her mother, or as her father's mother if she takes after that side. Girls with the uncommon genetic disorder known as *Turner's syndrome* are particularly prone to losing their follicles at a young age. An absolute minimum of one thousand follicles is required to cause menstruation, and by then the likelihood of conceiving is zero.

Apart from age and heredity, other common causes of follicle loss are:

↞ Radiation, for instance from radiotherapy

↞ Chemotherapy (these first two are only likely in someone who has undergone cancer treatment)

↞ Toxins, specifically, poisons made by certain bacteria, including some strains of streptococcus

↞ Oophoritis, that is, inflammation of the ovary, a complication of mumps

↞ Smoking. *All* women who smoke experience a reduction in fertility, but they may have been highly fertile in the first place, especially in their younger years, and therefore may be able to conceive without much problem

MENOPAUSE OR ANEMIA?

As mentioned early in the chapter, a big problem with anemia during the menopausal years is that the two conditions can produce similar symptoms, in both cases wide-ranging, imprecise, and variable. This sets the stage for much potential confusion. A middle-aged woman experiencing one or more of the signs indicating anemia may assume she is merely approaching "the change"—and so may her physician.

Some of the signs common to both anemia and perimenopause (the years approaching and encompassing menopause) include:

- Chronic fatigue

- Headaches

- Lack of concentration

- Feeling faint or dizzy

- Poor sleep

- Low or irritable mood

- Infertility

See Chapter 3 for a more detailed discussion of the signs and
symptoms of anemia.

Eleanor, encouraged by the example of the British prime min-
ister's wife, Cherie Blair, who gave birth at age forty-six,
was hopeful of becoming pregnant at a mere forty-two. But it
didn't prove that easy. She and her husband went through all
the fertility tests, but these failed to reveal any answers about
why she couldn't get pregnant. She felt it was too early to be
experiencing the change, and anyway she had none of the
characteristic menopausal symptoms, such as sweats and hot
flashes. In fact, her only complaints were of pins and needles
in her feet and one or two bouts of diarrhea, which seemed to
have no relation to anything. The bowel symptoms were put
down to diverticulitis—an important clue, as it turned out.

Diverticulitis can be associated with an overgrowth of bacteria in the intestines, which prevents the absorption of vitamin B-12. Another factor in Eleanor's case may have been her
habit of taking large doses of vitamin C, which interferes with
the body's ability to use vitamin B-12. Eleanor's doctor ran
through the blood tests again in the hope of turning up something that was relevant to her infertility. This time Eleanor had

a low hemoglobin level and a borderline low number of red blood corpuscles, many of them oversize.

Eleanor was teetering on the edge of pernicious anemia, a type caused by an autoimmune absence of the intrinsic factor needed for making blood, and by a lack of vitamin B-12 (hydroxocobalamin). Often this type of anemia arises with no symptoms at all until it is well established. Infertility may be the first indication of anything wrong, but since this is common anyway at Eleanor's age, the connection usually goes unrecognized. Symptoms to look out for in B-12 anemia are a sore, beefy-red tongue; periodic diarrhea (as in Eleanor's case); and weight loss, even though the person looks well. The clincher is a blood test showing a reduced amount of vitamin B-12 in the serum. (See Chapters 5 and 6 for more about B-12-deficiency anemia and pernicious anemia.)

Eleanor is receiving injections of B-12, and she remains hopeful that she may yet become pregnant.

PERIMENOPAUSE

Perimenopause encompasses the years leading up to menopause, as well as the shorter readjustment following a woman's very last menstrual period, lasting about six months. It typically begins in the early forties, as it did for Eleanor, when there has already been a substantial reduction in the number of follicles, including their granulosa cells, and a reduced output of estrogen and inhibin. Inhibin—although less important than estrogen in general—is useful in judging how many follicles still remain and how near a woman is to reaching menopause. A decrease in inhibin triggers an increase in FSH, follicular stimulating hormone. This is the body's desperate attempt to stimulate the flagging ovaries to release any available eggs—that is, a last shot at pregnancy. The amount of FSH in the blood fluctuates during the early forties and remains high, signifying that a woman is in the perimenopause. Conception at this point is unlikely; Cherie Blair was especially lucky.

One's FSH level gives a clear indication of the situation, but estrogen levels are less informative. Although the granulosa cells produce less estrogen during the perimenopause, compensatory arrangements take over to some extent and the typical menopausal symptoms are delayed several years. The ovaries continue to produce a little estrogen, but they also produce extra androgens (male-type hormones). These are converted into a weak form of estrogen, called *estrone*, by the liver and also by the fat cells, one bonus of being plump (i.e., menopausal symptoms may be delayed or lessened somewhat by a higher than normal output of estrone). The adrenal glands also manufacture testosterone (male hormone) and convert some of it into estrogen.

The increased quantities of androgens produced during perimenopause tend to cause a slight increase in facial hair and a loss of head hair. If a woman puts on weight, instead of its going to the hips and thighs in the typical feminine contour, it tends to stay in the abdomen, creating an apple shape instead of a pear shape. This body shape corresponds to a greater tendency for the arteries to clog up, making women as susceptible to heart attack as men. Another important reason to keep one's weight down is the greater risk overweight women run of developing cancer of the uterus or ovary. A woman 20 to 30 pounds overweight runs three times the risk of these cancers, while a 50-pound surplus increases her risk nine times. As well as being good for one's appearance and self-esteem, it can be life saving to keep a slim figure. (See the table on page 121 for ideal weight-to-height ratios once a woman reaches menopause.)

The diet, trimmed to achieve a reasonable weight, should consist of over 50 percent of calories from carbohydrate, around 15 percent from protein, and enough fat and sugar to make it all taste appetizing. The special nutrients it must provide include the minerals calcium and iron, and the vitamins C, D, and E, plus the B group, including folic acid.

Anemia During Perimenopause

As discussed elsewhere in this book, our bodies absorb only about 10 percent of the iron we consume in our diet. That's why, for menstruating women, the recommended iron intakes are so much higher than they are for men: 15 to 18 milligrams daily for a woman (depending on her age) versus 10 milligrams for a man. The leading cause of anemia is blood loss; therefore, when a woman's menstrual periods are fluctuating wildly, as they often do during perimenopause, when she might experience especially heavy bleeding, it is essential that she get her recommended daily intake of iron. Heme iron (that is, iron from animal sources such as meat, liver, and poultry) is absorbed much more readily by the human body than nonheme iron (which comes from plant sources such as green leafy vegetables). Vitamin C aids the absorption of all dietary iron.

But as Eleanor's case, above, demonstrates, although iron deficiency is the most common cause of anemia, it is not the only cause. Shortages and/or malabsorption of two of the B vitamins—B-12 and folic acid—can also lead to certain forms of anemia. Again, for a woman approaching menopause, awareness and vigilance are key to preventing or detecting anemia of any type.

THE DECADE OF MENOPAUSE

Ages forty-five to fifty-five are the menopausal years, with the LMP (last menstrual period) usually occurring between ages forty-nine and fifty-one. The decade of menopause brings with it special issues relating to a woman's body and her health, each of which can be complicated by untreated anemia lurking in her system, and each of which can be accompanied by special risk factors for anemia.

Ideal Weight for Height at Menopause

4′ 11″	108 to 129 lbs., depending on build (medium build 117 lbs.)
5′ 0″	109 to 132
5′ 1″	114 to 135
5′ 2″	117 to 139
5′ 3″	120 to 143
5′ 4″	124 to 147
5′ 5″	128 to 151
5′ 6″	132 to 155
5′ 7″	136 to 159
5′ 8″	141 to 164
5′ 9″	145 to 169
5′ 10″	149 to 175

Hysterectomy

If a woman has had a hysterectomy—that is, removal of the uterus—without the removal of the ovaries, menopause is likely to happen about two years earlier than normal. The removal of a woman's ovaries results in an instant or sudden menopause, sometimes called a *surgical menopause*, often with particularly severe symptoms, unless she is on hormone replacement.

Hysterectomy is now the most common major surgery in both the UK and the United States. In the UK one hundred thousand women annually (about thirty-five per ten thousand) undergo a hysterectomy, while in the U.S. a massive eight hundred thousand (about sixty-five per ten thousand) do so. Most hysterectomies are carried out at around age fifty; by age fifty-five at least 20 percent of women in the UK and 40 percent in the States have lost their wombs.

Jennifer developed a clutch of fibroids during her forties. These are noncancerous tumors of the uterus, made of fibrous tissue. Often they cause no problems, but in Jennifer's case they led to abnormally heavy periods, termed menorrhagia, which can lead to anemia. In the UK, the common disorder of fibroid tumors costs the government-run health service seven million pounds a year; in the U.S., by contrast, women with fibroids more often take the shortcut of a hysterectomy. Since hormonal treatment proved ineffective for Jennifer, and she was becoming increasingly anemic, her gynecologist advised her to have the operation.

It turned out that Jennifer was also anemic, a condition that would be important to correct before the surgery, when she was bound to lose more blood. Since treating her anemia with oral supplements would have taken weeks, she was given a transfusion as a flying start to restoring her blood to full strength. The happy ending for Jennifer was that after her hysterectomy she looked better and felt stronger and fitter than she had at any time in the last three or four years, ever since the excessive bleeding began.

Endometriosis

Endometriosis is an increasingly prevalent disorder in which patches of tissue identical to the lining of the uterus—and with the same propensity to bleed periodically—develop in and around the pelvic cavity. The bleeding caused by endometriosis increases a woman's risk of anemia from blood loss.

The most common symptom of endometriosis is pain at the site of the endometrial tissue, including deep pain during intercourse, called *dyspareunia*. Hormone treatment or surgery, including hysterectomy, may be called for, but if the patient can wait, menopause will come to the rescue. As menstrual periods stop, the abnormal tissue disappears.

Loss of Fertility

The very word *uterus* conjures up special emotional connotations. To have one's uterus surgically removed just at the time when she is entering menopause and thereby losing the ability to give birth can seem like locking the door and throwing away the key. While a woman still has a uterus she can fantasize in a private corner of her mind that a one in a thousand chance will come through and she will find herself pregnant. Once the organ is gone, so is the dream.

Susannah married late. When she and George tied the knot she was forty-one and her FSH level was already increasing, presaging the gradual shutdown of her reproductive function. She bravely dealt with the monthly disappointment of not finding herself pregnant, but when she developed endometriosis and had to have a hysterectomy she felt her life was over. Now she could no longer pretend, even to herself, that there was the slightest possibility of becoming a mother.

Susannah slipped through a sad mood into a clinical depression. She did not care about anyone or anything, neglected her appearance, could not sleep, and lost her appetite. She withdrew from all social activities and almost never left the house. A modern antidepressant related to Prozac, combined with six sessions of psychotherapy, enabled her to face life again and to gradually rediscover pleasures and satisfactions with her friends and loved ones.

Had the depression dragged on, Susannah would have been at risk of developing a physical illness—including anemia, partly because she wasn't eating properly, and partly due to the lack of emotional stimulus to make new blood, or new anything.

Other Risks

Other disorders that are prone to develop or become a nuisance during the decade of menopause—and to take precautions against—include:

   ⬧ Osteoporosis, a secondary effect of a low estrogen level. To avoid excessive bone loss, it is important to get plenty of calcium in your diet; good sources include skim milk, low-fat yogurt, Cheddar cheese, almonds, sardines or herring, and dried figs. The other half of the prescription is regular, weight-bearing exercise, at least forty minutes three times a week

↞ High blood pressure and coronary heart disease. Preventive tactics include taking calcium, but more important are cutting out extra sodium and animal fats, quitting smoking (the younger the better), maintaining a healthy weight, and keeping alcohol intake down to one drink a day

↞ Diabetes. Avoid eating too many sweets and too much fat

↞ Cancers. Antioxidants and plant foods, especially wheat and soy, are protective against cancer, while an excess of animal fats and meat seems to increase the risk. Exercise also has protective benefits. Smoking, on the other hand, is almost a sure cause of cancer

↞ Underactive thyroid (hypothyroidism). This is another disorder of the middle years especially, and it is on the increase. Like anemia, it comes on imperceptibly, but the late-stage results are dry, puffy skin; thinning hair, with loss of the outer third of the eyebrows; and a mild increase in weight. There is a general slowdown, both physical and mental. It is unpreventable, but treatment with daily thyroxine tablets is easy and effective

↞ Osteoarthritis, the disease marked by degeneration of the cartilage and bone in the joints. Regular exercise, short of straining, helps to ward it off, and so does moderating protein and alcohol intake. The anti-inflammatory drugs (NSAIDs) commonly used to treat osteoarthritis, including over-the-counter remedies such as ibuprofen, can cause bleeding ulcers in the stomach—which can lead to anemia from blood loss

Sheila was sixty. She had suffered with the nagging pain of osteoarthritis for several years, but not the type that could be relieved by hip replacement—it was in her back. She used various painkillers and NSAIDs (nonsteroidal anti-inflammatory drugs), some of them bought over the counter, so her doctor did not realize how much medication she was taking. One morning a disaster struck, seemingly out of the blue. Sheila woke up feeling sick and vomited nearly half a pint of blood, frightening herself and her husband. She was whisked off to the hospital, where she was given a blood transfusion—and her medication was overhauled. The NSAIDs had been most effective for controlling her pain, but they had caused tiny ulcers in the lining of her stomach, which had been leaking blood continuously. An excess of blood had built up in her stomach overnight.

A medicine known as an H2 blocker, such as ranitidine (Zantac) or cimetidine (Tagamet), was added to Sheila's medication to protect her stomach. To zap any tendency toward anemia she also now takes an iron tablet twice a week and makes sure to eat foods that provide iron—bran cereal, sardines, red meat, and dark chocolate—plus vitamin C, contained in fruits and vegetables, to help iron absorption.

PSYCHOSOCIAL ASPECTS OF MENOPAUSE

A hundred and fifty years ago menopause was dreaded. It was reputed to cause madness, "often called forth a sense of religion" in an era when God was more a god of vengeance than one of love, and promoted "habits of intoxication" through poverty and poor education. Great play was made of the waning of personal beauty, although "the desire of pleasing was undiminished." This conflicting situation caused, the doctors said, jealousy and depression, even suicide. (From Quain, *Dictionary of Medicine,* 1885.)

Today the situation is almost the reverse. The menopausal years can be a time of rejuvenation. They are certainly among the most interesting of a woman's life, appropriately full of change. If you are a career woman you may be just a fingertip away from the top job, or you may be celebrating your recent escape from the kitchen, the house, and looking after young children—much as you love them. Now is your chance to write that novel, go on a safari, or even return to college. You are young enough to do anything you set your mind to, but old enough to have garnered a wealth of experience that will keep you safely on track.

Menopause is a major life event in itself, and there are other social and emotional hurdles you may have to clear at the same time. One is the "empty nest syndrome" that frequently occurs when your youngest child leaves home. You are better off if you already have an outside job, but in any case now is a good time to reinforce your same-age friendships—and to branch out into new activities: to join a writers' circle, take a computer course, or form a golf, bridge, or theater club.

Marital misery and/or divorce may raise their undesirable heads at this time, when you are already feeling emotional. Men do not undergo menopause, but they tend to cling to the remains of their youth as they enter their fifties. A new, younger mate may seem like the answer. Your man's "midlife crisis" is a phase that may pass, but in any event it makes sense for you to build your own independent life.

Other common "new" problems might involve your parents. It is disconcerting to find that you and they are trading roles. You can no longer rely on being able to turn to the older generation—they will soon be leaning on you. This is only fair: They changed your diapers when you were too young to care for yourself.

Illness and death may affect those you love, although now that we live so much longer it comes as a shock when a parent in his or her seventies, eighties, or nineties dies. A parent's death may not be a tragedy if you view it rationally, but it is bound to give you a jolt, and it is important to allow yourself whatever time and space you need to grieve these losses. The passing of the older generation reminds you that your generation is now the first in line. This can be quite a chilling thought when you first realize it, but at your age you potentially still have decades to look forward to.

The main message of menopause is that now is the time to take charge of your own life—and especially of your health, both physical and psychological. Sidestepping the physical and behavioral problems that accompany anemia—the disconcerting lethargy, irritability, insomnia, and loss of concentration—will only enhance your feelings of energy, happiness, and empowerment during these newly free years. Doing so involves three steps. First, learn and follow the strategies for preventing anemia provided throughout this book. Second, acquaint yourself with the signs and symptoms of anemia, spelled out in this chapter and in more detail in Chapters 3 through 7. Third, if you experience one or more of the warning signs for anemia, don't be guilty of writing them off as inevitable "age-related changes" or "side effects of menopause." They may not be. If you're not feeling yourself, pay a visit to your health-care professional and request to be evaluated for anemia.

Welcome the challenges of this time of your life in the best health you can achieve. Isn't it good to feel that you are captain of the ship?

12

The Senior Years

The senior years are at last being recognized as definite life stages, with their own particular characteristics, problems, and needs. Called the *third and fourth ages* in the UK, these years cover from ages sixty-five to eighty (the "third age"), and over age eighty (the "fourth age"). Both are risk periods for anemia. You might think that when a person is neither growing nor undergoing some major bodily upheaval such as pregnancy or menopause, she would be past any danger of anemia. Wrong. Twenty percent of women as young as age sixty are anemic even in the well-fed West, and the proportion increases year by year as we get older.

The insidious way anemia can creep up and catch someone unawares is illustrated by the case of the British Queen Mother. Although she was probably the most cosseted and cared-for old lady in England, in 2001 she had to be rushed into the hospital—for anemia. Her leading symptom was a feeling of exhaustion—understandable at her age, 101—and at first it was put down to an unexpected heat wave.

WHAT MAKES OLDER PEOPLE ESPECIALLY VULNERABLE?

The two main causes of anemia at any age are an inadequate intake of nourishment and a loss of blood, most often through a slow leak. Bleeding hemorrhoids were thought to be the cause of the Queen Mother's anemia. But for many older people, poor nutrition is the culprit. One major factor in this problem is living alone, which has an effect on the types of foods a person eats. A huge proportion of women over age sixty-five live alone, many of them widows, since men pass away on average seven years earlier than their partners.

> Edna was seventy-three when her husband Arthur died. It caused a revolution in her lifestyle when she no longer had a man to feed. Arthur had liked the full works—a cooked breakfast of bacon and eggs, a midday meal with meat and vegetables and something sweet for dessert, and a supper of beans, sardines, or herring on toast, plus a bedtime drink of hot chocolate with cake or cookies. Arthur never ran short of calories or iron, and neither did Edna when he was alive.
>
> Of course, she missed him dreadfully, even his bad temper, but she found it a relief not having to cook all the time. Her meals became progressively simpler, with meat and vegetables going by the wayside first. Toast or a scone with jam or honey, or a bowl of porridge or cold cereal replaced the more complicated dishes, washed down with plenty of good strong tea. If she still felt hungry there was always a cookie or a slice of cake to fill the cracks.
>
> The downside was her slide into anemia. Since she was not an outdoor person Edna had always had a pale complexion, so this symptom was not particularly significant, but her increasing weakness and weariness were a direct result of a shortage of hemoglobin. She was not eating enough of the protein necessary to make hemoglobin. She was short of iron, also required for hemoglobin. Both protein and iron are best supplied by meat or liver, neither of which she bothered with now

that Arthur was not there to demand them. The numerous cups of tea Edna enjoyed had the effect of inhibiting the absorption of the small amount of iron that was in her food. Similarly, her favorite breakfast of porridge contained phytates, which have the same effect as black tea on inhibiting iron absorption.

Hemoglobin is the special protein that makes blood red and carries oxygen to the muscles, nerves, and brain. A lack of hemoglobin is the essence of anemia, and it was the condition that was siphoning off all of Edna's energy, muscle strength, and powers of concentration. Myoglobin, a protein contained in muscle, also requires iron and protein in its manufacture; an insufficient supply of it accounted for some of Edna's weakness.

A complete reorganization of Edna's diet and lifestyle—plus more or less indefinite supplementation with liquid iron, which avoided the indigestion that bothered her with iron tablets—gave her a new lease of energy.

Poor Appetite

Some older people simply fail to eat enough. It is normal and natural to eat less as one gets older and becomes less active, but this trend may carry a person too far and land her in a vicious circle. She may get very little exercise because of arthritis or a temporary problem like a cold, so she feels less hungry. She eats less and then lacks the energy to go for a healthy walk—and the downward spiral continues.

Appetite can also be severely diminished by certain medicines, for example, glucagon, morphine and its derivatives such as codeine, phenylbutazone, salbutamol, indomethacin, levodopa, and several heart medicines. A few, such as penicillamine, make everything taste peculiar.

Cigarettes not only kill one's appetite but also impair digestion.

Poor Absorption

As do tannin-containing beverages such as coffee and black tea, some drugs interfere with the absorption of iron in particular—for example, antacids, such as those found in indigestion tablets, and tetracycline. Taking them increases the risk of iron-deficiency anemia. By contrast, ascorbic acid (vitamin C), citric acid, fructose (fruit sugar), and lactic acid (milk sugar) increase the absorption of iron. An orange a day is a useful prophylactic. Additionally, older people simply do not digest meat (or other foods) as efficiently. This phenomenon is due to an age-related decrease in the production of stomach acid, which contains digestive enzymes.

OTHER FOOD SUBSTANCES NEEDED TO PREVENT ANEMIA

Besides iron, other nutrients are necessary to prevent specific types of anemia. These include the following:

Vitamin B-12, available only in animal foods. Its absorption is reduced by slow-release potassium, cimetidine, ranitidine, trifluoperazine, an excess of vitamin C—and smoking. B-12 is freely available in meat, sardines, cheese, eggs, and liver. Vegetarians are most at risk for B-12-deficiency anemia.

Folate (folic acid). Absorption of this B vitamin is counteracted by alcohol, phenytoin, cholestyramine, and the anti-cancer drug methotrexate. A lack of folate is the most common vitamin deficiency among hospital patients in Western countries. The chief food sources are liver, fortified breakfast cereals, soy, wheat germ, sprouts and other green vegetables, lettuce, fruit, whole-grain bread, and eggs. Asian women who rely excessively on rice are the most likely to develop anemia from lack of folate.

SYMPTOMS OF ANEMIA THAT ARE EASILY MISSED IN THE ELDERLY

When a person's blood is lacking in hemoglobin, the oxygen carrier, his or her heart has to pump harder to make the blood circulate more quickly. This in turn causes the following symptoms, easy to miss in the elderly because they may be written off as the consequences of old age! (See also Chapters 3 through 7 for detailed lists of symptoms related to specific types of anemia.)

+ Getting winded easily—it's especially difficult to walk and talk, especially going uphill

+ Swollen ankles

+ Angina—pain in the chest while performing a little exercise, such as walking

+ Weak muscles—everything becomes an effort

+ Headaches

Something seniors need *not* worry about are those red, then purple and brownish spots that sometimes appear on the skin of the hands and forearms or other areas subject to mild daily wear and tear. These are harmless reminders of maturity. As we age, the walls of the smallest blood vessels lose elasticity, allowing a little leakage. The macrophages—cells that clear away old or broken red blood cells—are slower to respond than they were at age twenty-one, so these tiny hemorrhages take a long time to disappear.

Another normal change is a lower level of hemoglobin in the blood. It decreases a little starting at age sixty, and even more sharply at seventy, because of the body's less-demanding metabolism. A hemoglobin level anywhere above 10 g/dl (grams per deciliter) is perfectly acceptable at age seventy-plus and does not spell anemia.

Breathe Easier

If you do get winded and feel weak easily, or if you do have angina, *and if your doctor has ruled out anemia*, try the following health-enhancing suggestions:

✦ Breathe deeply. Of course you must give up smoking, if you are old-fashioned enough to still be doing it, but even for nonsmokers it is beneficial to take a few deep breaths every morning and evening—to open up the bottom corners of the lungs. Stand tall and walk tall so as to avoid cramping the chest, and shed a pound or two if your breathing—and thus your oxygenation— is impeded by a layer of fat. A gentle daily walk is good for the heart and chest, even if you have angina. Angina usually responds well to a glyceryl trinitrate (GTN) tablet under the tongue

✦ Shut your windows tight against fog or mist, and don't be a fresh-air fiend in winter. Don't go to bed in a cold room—warm it first, and air your bedroom during the day

The relevant dietary suggestions for heart and circulation problems include:

✦ Keeping protein intake up

✦ Keeping salt intake down

RED ALERT FOR PEOPLE OVER SEVENTY

If you are seventy or older, you are special. Ordinary rules don't apply. Your body, to make things easy for you, is adjusting to suit retirement-type activities. You want to feel 100 percent fit, but you won't be aiming to beat the Williams sisters at tennis or to out-throw Dan Marino on the football field. It is only sensible to scale back on the athletics and concentrate on the areas where your interests now lie.

Your body will shift gears into a more economical mode; play along with it for maximum benefit. For example, why waste resources on producing pigment for your hair when it looks just as elegant in white or gray at this age? For women, it would be crazy to go on pouring out hormones in an endless rhythm of blood-wasting menstrual periods on the off chance of your wanting a baby at this stage in life. And most men have surely advanced past the need for arduous manual labor. There is no call at this stage of the game for either sex to carry a heavy skeleton and powerful muscles, when lighter equipment will serve.

On the other hand your heart isn't fazed by your age, and barring accidents or ill health it can go on beating steadily into the nineties and beyond. However, it may take a moment or two longer for your circulation to adjust when you get up from a low chair, and although your lungs will easily take in all the oxygen you need for ordinary living, it will take a little more effort to sing or to make a speech.

Your Blood

Blood is affected by the normal changes in your digestive system. Your stomach will be making slightly less acid, and this means that certain substances are less well absorbed. These include some of the essentials for making blood: iron and vitamins B-12 and C. You may also produce a little less intrinsic factor, the substance that enables your body to absorb vitamin B-12. These changes mean that you must make sure to eat your daily orange or its equivalent to supply your body with vitamin C; meat, preferably red, two or three times a week for vitamin B-12; and other protein foods such as cheese, fish, chicken, and eggs (lentils and other beans, especially soy, provide some protein, but nuts may be too difficult to digest). Remember—you need almost as much protein at seventy-five as you did at thirty-five, and vegetables for the folic acid they provide.

Failure to get enough iron is a common problem for people in this age bracket: Up to 20 percent of those over seventy have iron-deficiency anemia, and thus feel tired unnecessarily. The reduction in stomach acid is one factor, but the other is up to you. Because your teeth may be less efficient than when you were younger, it is less trouble to eat a bun or a cookie than it is to cut up some fruit to eat. But you need the vitamin C in the fruit to help you make the most of the iron in your food. Dairy products, too, help the absorption of iron, through the calcium they contain.

The foods that supply iron include meat, liver, bran cereal, dark chocolate, and oatmeal. Porridge is an excellent provider of iron, but you must take milk with it, to neutralize the phytic acid.

You may feel that you now need smaller meals than when you were younger; however, be sure that you don't cut down on the nutrients necessary to produce blood. Instead, you can safely reduce your intake of fillers such as cookies, cakes, potatoes, rice, bread, and pasta.

Once you reach your eighties or nineties, you can afford to relax. You know you have a first-class constitution, or you would not still be here, and you need not worry about restricting your cholesterol or becoming overweight. Your emphasis should be on enjoying your food and your family, and on getting plenty of grains, vegetables, and fruit.

Expect to lose height as well as some of the padding of fat just under the skin. This is normal, but you must make sure to keep warm, and to have a cushion to sit on for comfort.

Congratulations on having arrived in the top class!

Chapter

13

How to Avoid Anemia

Keeping healthy is not usually much fun: It involves tedious and tiring exercise, freezing-cold temperatures, coating your skin with sunscreen when it is sunny and warm outside, and remembering your posture when your instinct is to slump. The delightful truth about the steps you should take to sidestep anemia, however, is that they are enjoyable. They involve eating enough good food to ensure that you have plenty of the healthy blood-forming nutrients—the opposite of the usual wearisome diet routine, for women at least, of feeling guilty about eating almost anything. Since we may absorb as little as 10 percent of our intake of some nutrients, we must eat enough and some to spare of the vital ingredients of an anti-anemia diet: protein, iron, and the vitamins B-12, C, and folic acid. Calcium is useful, too; it helps in the absorption of iron.

PROTEIN

Since the -*globin* part of hemoglobin is itself a protein, eating plenty of high-quality protein is a must for manufacturing high-quality blood and preventing anemia. Proteins are composed of various amino acids. There are twenty-two of these, of which nine are called *essential*. They comprise lysine, methionine, phenylalanine, leucine, threonine, tryptophan, valine, isoleucine, and histidine. We must get all nine of these from the foods we eat. The other thirteen amino acids are called *nonessential*—not because our body doesn't need them, but because we can manufacture them from the other nine.

Not all protein in foods is created equal. With the exception of soy, the protein contained in any single plant food—for example, grains, beans, peas, or nuts—does not contain all nine of the essential amino acids; therefore, the protein provided by these foods is called *incomplete*. The combination of grains and beans provides some of each of the essential amino acids. Carefully combining foods—that is, consuming adequate portions of both grains and beans every day—is one way for vegetarians to get complete protein in their diet. Eating several servings of soy every day is another way. Soy is the only plant food that contains all nine essential amino acids. Otherwise, meat—as well as other foods that come from animal sources, such as eggs and dairy products—provides all the essential amino acids. Meat also provides another essential nutrient, unavailable in reliable amounts from any plant source, including soy: vitamin B-12. Combining grains and beans might give you complete protein, but it won't give you vitamin B-12. Additionally, the mixture of grains and beans is only about 13 percent protein, so a person would have to eat a huge amount of these foods to supply all the protein he or she needs.

The plant foods that contain some protein are the following:

The most: soy, legumes (dried peas and beans), and nuts

Some: brown bread, brown rice, and corn

Negligible: bananas and potatoes

It is recommended that women consume about 60 grams of protein daily. The absolute minimum is 40 grams, and that must be first-class stuff: the kind available in meat, fish, poultry, eggs, hard cheese, and soy. Protein should make up 10 to 20 percent of a person's total caloric intake. Children, pregnant and breast-feeding women, and men doing exceptionally heavy work need proportionately more—maybe double. And we all need extra protein for repair work to our tissues or following a loss of blood from any cause—be it an illness, an injury, or a burn. Babies get their protein, like they do everything else, from breast milk or formula.

Because of the importance of blood, the requirements of the blood factory in the bone marrow take priority over other body parts for any available protein. If protein supplies are meager, muscles and other organs may get short shrift. Rather alarmingly, they will waste away if their tissues remain unreplenished with new protein.

Those at risk of not obtaining enough protein include vegetarians who fail to carefully observe guidelines for obtaining complete protein, Asians who rely on a diet of vegetables and/or rice, and those in the special groups mentioned above.

Protein Content of Some Common Foods

Food	Serving size	Protein (grams)
Lean ground beef	3 oz.	21
Skim milk	8 fluid oz.	8.35
Whole egg (extra large)	1	7.2
Chicken, dark meat	3.5 oz.	27
Tuna, canned in water	4 oz.	29
Cheese, cheddar	1 oz.	7
Tofu (soybean curd), firm, raw	½ cup	20
Black-eyed peas, boiled	½ cup	20 (incomplete)
Rice, brown, cooked	1 cup	5 (incomplete)

IRON

Getting enough iron in the diet is vital for manufacturing the other half of hemoglobin—the heme molecule. Iron is the constituent of blood most likely to run short. It is available in the following foods:

Best sources: liver, corned beef, fresh beef and lamb, blackstrap molasses, oatmeal

Good sources: eggs, dark chocolate, peas, beans, bran cereal, bread, soy

Moderate sources: fish, milk, most nuts, fruits, root vegetables

Spinach, via Popeye, has a great reputation as a provider of iron, and indeed of the vegetables it is the best source of the mineral. The snag is that it takes quadruple servings of spinach to do much good, and the same goes for broccoli, cabbage, and sprouts. In any case, a normal mixed diet provides more iron than a vegetarian diet, and also enables the body to absorb the iron better. This is partly because, as discussed earlier in the book, the iron from plant sources (nonheme iron) is less readily absorbed by the body than the iron from animal sources (heme iron). Calcium, found in all kinds of dairy products, also helps iron absorption, as does vitamin C, from fresh fruit; by contrast, coffee, black tea, and the phytic acid in unmilled grains inhibit absorption.

The groups who require extra iron are the same as those needing extra supplies of protein; in addition, all menstruating women have a 5 percent deficit in their iron stores (from blood loss) to make up at all times.

VITAMIN B-12 AND FOLIC ACID

This is "the meat and vegetable partnership": two B-complex vitamins that function together in making blood, one that comes from meat and the other from vegetables. B-12 comes solely from animal sources; folic acid comes from plants and some animal products. Fruits, vegetables, bread, and grains are a waste of time as far as B-12 is concerned, while on the other hand fresh green vegetables, especially spinach and broccoli, are tops for providing folate (so is liver). (A reminder about good sources of folate is the fact that, by coincidence, the first part of the word *folate* is the same as the first part of the word *foliage*. Folic acid comes from foliage, or green leafy vegetables.) Whole-grain bread, bananas, beef, ham, and eggs are the next best sources of folate, but fruit, milk, lamb, pork, and poultry don't really register on the chart.

Our bodies carry a big reserve of B-12 against contingencies, so we don't need to eat B-12 foods every day; but we store only enough folate to last us for a few weeks, so it is wise to keep maximum supplies of this vitamin in our bodies. Again, those who are still growing, as well as the other needy groups, especially pregnant women, demand extra amounts of each of these vitamins.

VITAMIN C

There is no excuse for anyone to run low of this vitamin, since it abounds in such delicious foods as citrus fruits, berries, mangoes, and pineapple. Lettuces, other raw green vegetables, tomatoes, broccoli, and peppers are also first class for this vitamin. Apples, plums, cherries, pears, and melons rank second for vitamin C, while milk and meat are of no use.

DIETARY DON'TS

To ensure that you're getting the most from the foods you eat, pay attention to the following general guidelines:

✦ Don't wreck good food by unnecessary cooking. Heat wipes out most of the vitamin C and folates in a food. Raw is best, and lightly cooked is better than well cooked. Therefore, French fries are better, vitamin-wise (if not fat-content-wise), than boiled or roasted potatoes—the cooking time is shorter.

* Don't boil vegetables; steam them instead. Both iron and vitamins are lost in the water.

* Don't rely too heavily on oatmeal, whole wheat, and other unprocessed grains. These foods contain iron, but they are also full of phytic acid, which prevents the absorption of both iron and the useful mineral calcium.

* Don't drink too much coffee or black tea, and don't take them too strong. These beverages also inhibit the absorption of iron.

* Don't take iron pills with or after food. They are better absorbed if taken before a meal.

* Don't take iron pills at short intervals. There is a six-hour refractory period after each dose during which the body won't take in any more iron.

* Don't store fruits and vegetables out in the open. Exposure to air causes a loss of vitamin C.

* Don't bruise or cut fruit or salad greens until just before eating them. Vitamin C escapes from cut fruits and vegetables.

* Don't rely just on plant foods. Eat at least some cheese, eggs, milk, and fish, too, if possible. At the very minimum, a strict vegan diet needs to be supplemented with iron and vitamin B-12.

WATCH YOUR ALCOHOL INTAKE

Alcohol is one of life's pleasures that you need not miss out on, but like gambling it can be harmful if you indulge too much, especially if your taste runs to hard liquor. Substantial drinking can lead to anemia by several routes:

- A direct poisoning effect of alcohol on red blood cells and also on bone marrow. The red cells become oversize, even before anemia sets in

- Strain on the liver from having to deal with the alcohol, so that the liver cannot play its role properly in the metabolism of blood

- Inflammation of the digestive tract (think of the feeling of warmth as a mouthful of whisky or vodka goes down), leading to small, unnoticed hemorrhages and, in later stages, to large ones. Either way it means a loss of blood—and anemia

- Folate deficiency because of impaired metabolism

- A generally poor diet. A person may use a drink as a pick-me-up when she really needs a proper meal, and many drinkers lose their appetite (the thought of break-fast turns the stomach if someone is hung over)

- Alcoholic gastritis may interfere with the production in the stomach of the intrinsic factor, leading to pernicious anemia

COULD YOU BE LOSING BLOOD WITHOUT REALIZING IT?

Unnoticed blood loss is a very common cause of anemia; the leakage or seeping away of a teaspoonful of blood per day is enough to cause its onset. If you have any of the symptoms of anemia, consider whether bleeding due to any of these problems could be responsible:

✦ hemorrhoids

✦ hiatal hernia

✦ peptic ulcer

✦ diverticular disease (age-related changes in the colon)

✦ ulcerative colitis

✦ long, frequent, or heavy menstrual periods

✦ other gynecological problems such as endometriosis

✦ nosebleeds from infection or high blood pressure

IS IT IN YOUR GENES?

Find out the answers to the following questions regarding your family members:

✦ Do you have any relative with anemia?

✦ Do you have any relative with sickle-cell disorder?

✦ Is there any family tendency to autoimmune disorders? These include type-1 diabetes, vitiligo, rheumatoid arthritis, lupus, thyroid disorders, pernicious anemia, autoimmune gastritis, dermatomyositis, certain liver disorders, and Goodpasture's kidney disease.

Any of these conditions in you or a relative makes you more vulnerable to anemia. That means if the answer to any of these questions is "yes," you should be extra watchful for the early, vague symptoms of anemia—and, if in doubt, get your blood checked.

MEDICINES THAT MAY TRIGGER ANEMIA
(BUT USUALLY DO NOT)

Be vigilant about your use of the following medications, which can (but usually do not) trigger anemia:

- painkillers such as aspirin, phenacetin, and the non-steroidal anti-inflammatory drugs (NSAIDs) such as ibuprofen (Advil) used in joint and rheumatic pain

- steroids such as prednisolone

- gold, phenylbutazone (Butazolidin), isoniazid

- phenytoin (Epanutin), primodone, phenobarbital, sodium valproate

- oral contraceptives

- neomycin, metformin (Glucophage)

- penicillin, tetracycline, nitrofurantoin (Furadantin), sulfonamides

- carbimazole

- captopril, nifedipine (for high blood pressure)

- mood drugs: amitriptyline (Tryptizol), chlorpromazine, mianserin, clozapine, dothiepin

- quinidine, chlorpropamide

- Tagamet, Zantac

- dapsone, Salazopyrin

WARNING SIGNS

If you experience any of the following symptoms, make an appointment with your doctor, tell him or her about your suspicions, and ask to be checked for anemia:

* Weakness and weariness

* Unsteady walk

* Forgetfulness or confusion

* Loss of sensation or pins and needles in the feet and/or hands

* Sore tongue

SENSIBLE EATING

Besides getting plenty of the vital anemia-preventing nutrients discussed at the beginning of this chapter, a good overall diet is essential to an effective anti-anemia lifestyle.

Suggestions for Anti-Anemia Meals

Below are some sample menus that would constitute a diet well suited for preventing anemia. Add snacks and/or second helpings according to your appetite and caloric needs.

Note: Although the menus list coffee and tea as acceptable beverages, limit your consumption of these drinks to a maximum of two or three cups per day; more can inhibit the absorption of iron.

Breakfasts

Porridge or granola with honey and milk. Orange juice. Toast. Coffee or tea.

Grilled tomatoes or mushrooms on whole-grain toast. Coffee or tea.

Boiled, poached, or scrambled egg with toast and spread. Orange or other fruit. Coffee or tea.

Ham or bacon with tomatoes and toast. Coffee, tea, or juice.

Mixed fruits, bagel, and soft cheese. Coffee, tea, or juice.

Lunches

Sandwich on whole-grain bread, with cheese, ham or turkey or chicken, mustard and mayonnaise, lettuce and tomato. Piece of fruit. Yogurt. Coffee, hot chocolate, juice, or beer.

Baked potato with filling of meat, cheese, ham, tuna, or chicken, with a piece of fruit or salad. Beverage.

Meat, ham, egg, or cheese, with salad and a brown roll. Yogurt or apple pie. Beverage.

Suppers

Glass of wine (optional).

Four ounces of lean meat or the equivalent, with salad or raw or steamed vegetables, and a dairy product, e.g., yogurt, custard, or cheese.

Main Course

Braised liver, onions, and potatoes

Bean and vegetable curry with brown rice

Lamb chop, broccoli, carrots, and potatoes

Slice of steak, with onions, mushrooms, and tomatoes, plus roll

Stir-fried chicken and mixed vegetables, with flatbread

White fish, spinach, and fries

Roast beef or lamb, with green vegetables and potatoes

Omelet of bell peppers and tomatoes, with roll

Calories Needed		
Both sexes	0–1 year	800
	2–3	1,400
	5–7	1,800
Boys	9–12	2,500
	15–18	3,000
Girls	9–12	2,300
	15–18	2,300
Men	18–55	2,700–3,600
	60+	1,900
Women	18–55	2,200
	in pregnancy	2,400
	60+	1,700

The calorie levels presented above are a general guideline. You need more or fewer calories according to your size and the amount of energy you use. For instance, serious athletes or those who perform heavy manual labor need more; those who are small-framed or who get little to no exercise need fewer.

Dessert

Baked apple with raisins and ice cream

Fruit pie

Egg custard and stewed fruit

Grilled grapefruit and chocolate cookie

Cheese with apple or crackers

Fruit sorbet, cookie

Raspberry mousse

Baked banana

Fresh fruit at any time

A Note for Babies

Babies must begin eating mixed solid foods by the time they are four months old. Start with purees of vegetables and fruits, and a month or so later try purees with some meat incorporated. Starting at age eight months, minced food is manageable, and starting at one year eggs are very useful. Starting from age six months fruit juice should replace milk as the drink to accompany meals.

Parents need to introduce vegetable purees early, because from around age three to four months a baby may run short of iron; even the very best breast milk or formula does not supply enough. Babies adapt to strange-tasting foods more easily at younger than five months than they do later. From toddler stage onwards a child can digest most of the foods parents have at home, but he or she is still susceptible to choking on hard pieces and lumps until age two and a half or three years.

It is in childhood that healthy eating habits are learned—habits that will last a lifetime. As an adult you are responsible for developing your own good habits. Bon appetit!

14

Herbal Medicines
and Anemia

Herbal medicines can be useful in treating iron-deficiency anemia and, to a lesser extent, B-12-deficiency anemia. The science
of herbal medicine has been practiced for thousands of years by
all civilizations, but its prominence in Western culture has faded
significantly over the last couple of centuries with the development of modern medicine. Even so, the constituents of medicinal plants are still contained in the active ingredients of many
modern drugs (although nowadays, rather than extracting these
ingredients from actual plants, manufacturers of pharmaceuti-
cals may create synthetic versions of them in the chemistry lab).
Some common examples include aspirin (whose active ingredient, salicylic acid, derives from the medicinal herb white willow
bark) and certain cold/allergy remedies that contain the ingredient ephedrine or pseudoephedrine (which comes from the herb
ephedra, or ma huang). But medicinal herbs don't just include
exotic plants. Common fruits and vegetables—such as spinach,
garlic, and wild strawberry—can also be used therapeutically.

Herbal medicine is regaining popularity in the West as
people realize that it is a relatively inexpensive and effective
therapy. And many users of herbal medicines like the fact that

the ingredients come directly from nature. However, just because they're "natural," and just because they're nonprescription, herbal remedies shouldn't be utilized carelessly. They are powerful medicines in their own right, with side effects that can be serious. Their use must be undertaken conscientiously. Especially if you take any prescription medication, discuss your planned use of herbal preparations with your health-care practitioner. At the very least, follow the remedy's label instructions carefully, especially with regard to dosage, just as you would with any over-the-counter medicine. Don't make the mistaken assumption that just because some is good, more must be better.

The easiest place to obtain herbal medicines is from natural-food stores, but regular drugstores now stock these products more often as they grow increasingly popular. Good brands are also available through direct-marketing companies, as well as over the Internet. Some herbs can be grown at home, but extracting the vital ingredients is often tricky and time-consuming. It is usually ineffective to simply pluck a few plants from the ground and brew them into a tea; to obtain the most benefit from a medicinal plant, its health-promoting ingredients must be "standardized" to a specific concentration.

The herbal treatment of anemia is generally pleasant and free of side effects, but it acts slowly and uncertainly. Moreover, such remedies require supplementing if vitamin B-12 is the deficient nutrient, since B-12 is found in reliable amounts only in animal sources. Most sufferers of severe cases of anemia will need to undergo conventional therapy first—such as a blood transfusion or B-12 injections—perhaps followed up with an herbal treatment to maintain optimum blood health.

IRON-DEFICIENCY ANEMIA

By far the most common kind of anemia is iron-deficiency anemia, and naturally the main treatment for it is increasing one's intake of iron. Extra iron is also necessary for prevention of anemia in vulnerable groups such as pregnant women, fast-growing babies and adolescents, and the elderly. (See Chapters 8 through 12 for individual discussion of these various life stages.)

Cheap, commercially produced iron-supplement tablets are readily available from pharmacies and drugstores, usually in the form of an iron salt such as ferrous sulfate. The trouble with iron tablets, as discussed earlier in the book, is that side effects such as an upset stomach and bowels are very common; in some individuals these effects are so severe that they find it impossible to take iron tablets. For such patients in particular herbal iron preparations are useful—as well as for anyone wanting to avoid even the mild side effects potentially caused by conventional iron tablets. An added advantage of the herbal medicines is that the iron is often better absorbed than it is from conventional iron tablets.

Natural sources of iron include a variety of plants, especially ocean kelp and other seaweeds, stinging nettles, couch grass root, gotu kola (Asian pennywort), and parsley. Less rich in iron—but still effective enough to be considered as remedies—are burdock, devil's claw, silverweed, spinach, toadflax, wild strawberry, meadowsweet, and mullein.

Floradix brand herbal iron extract, made by the German company Salus-Haus, is a supplement containing organic iron from a mixture of herbs, including mallow, yarrow, carrots, fennel, and angelica root, with wormwood as an aid to digestion, juniper berries to boost the metabolism, and hawthorn as a tonic to the heart. The iron is prepared with the use of yeast, which incorporates the mineral into its cells.

Practitioners of herbal medicine advise their iron-deficient patients to avoid substances that inhibit iron absorption, such as chocolate, egg yolk, coffee, black tea, and wheat bran, as well as indigestion mixtures (such as Tagamet), tetracyclines (a form of antibiotic), phosphates (such as sodium phosphate, used in enemas), phytates (found in oatmeal and whole-grain cereals), and an excess of supplemental calcium. Recommended vitamins include vitamin C especially (because it enhances iron absorption), as well as vitamin B-12 and folic acid. For prevention of iron deficiency, it is excellent practice for anyone to incorporate in their diet the plants and herbal teas containing iron.

The symptoms of anemia most likely to respond to herbal remedies are tiredness, dizziness, palpitations, shortness of breath, and finding any activity a struggle. Herbs that a have a specific effect on these symptoms—more as general stimulants than as sources of iron—include echinacea (Black Sampson), hops, nettles, red clover, motherwort, barberry, and dandelion.

Edwina was a fitness freak, indulging in tai chi, transcendental meditation, running, and regular sessions at the gym under the guidance of her personal trainer. By rights, at twenty-seven, she should have been a bundle of energy and have taken her pregnancy in stride. To her puzzlement and chagrin she found that she was lagging behind the others at the prenatal class and was distinctly short of breath. Instead of seeing more results when she tried harder and put more effort into her training, she simply felt more depleted and exhausted.

Her doctor, a big, beefy fellow, who did no more muscle work than was necessary to lift a glass, patted her arm and told her not to worry. More to the point, he sent her blood sample for a full count. It turned out that Edwina had severe iron-deficiency anemia. The treatment—daily iron tablets, could not have been simpler, her doctor said breezily. That was in theory. The snag was that Edwina's body could not tolerate the medication, whether coated tablets or the liquid preparations. They gave her stomachaches and loose bowel movements from Day One.

She lost faith in her doctor and sought out an alternative therapist who directed her to a herbalist colleague. The new treatment involved eating large amounts of iron-containing vegetables such as spinach, watercress, and parsley and a cocktail of herbs, including mugwort and gentian. Echinacea was added, since it has a reputation for stimulating the production of red blood cells.

The mild herbal medicine gradually corrected Edwina's lack of iron, and her body and her mind were again working with full energy. Edwina made sure that her baby, the innocent cause of her original lack of iron, had feeds and purees fortified with iron from the age of five months. She and her child were prize winners in a beautiful mother and baby competition.

ANEMIA ASSOCIATED WITH A LACK OF B-12, INCLUDING PERNICIOUS ANEMIA

Vitamin B-12 is obtainable in reliable amounts only from animal products, which presents a problem for committed vegetarians and, especially, vegans. Whatever plants and herbs and nuts they eat, they must also get injections of the vitamin or take supplements. Plants that are palatable and possibly useful include comfrey and Icelandic moss; these are sometimes made into a puree with garlic. Others are milk thistle, centaury, blue flag, yellow dock, and red clover.

Aileen was fifty-five, an animal lover, and a vegetarian on principle. One of her favorite quotes was that of George Bernard Shaw, comparing the power in an acorn that can develop into a mighty oak tree with a slice of rump steak that gives you one meal and is finished. Aileen ate a lot of vegetables—including those rich in iron, also a variety of beans, especially soy, and nuts, seeds, and wholegrain, to supply plant proteins.

She would have gotten by in good health, without touching meat or other animal food, if it had not been for the bleeding fibroids. They started to become troublesome with the onset of her menopause. Now she showed the nonspecific signs and symptoms of anemia, plus a sore tongue and faintly yellow complexion that marked it out as the megaloblastic type. This develops when there is a lack of vitamin B-12. Usually this is due to pernicious anemia, an autoimmune disorder, but in

Aileen's case it was because the blood loss from the fibroids had used up all her vitamin B-12 reserves.

Neither Aileen's comprehensive vegetarian diet nor the herbal and dietary treatment for iron deficiency anemia suggested for Edwina was enough to restore her health and energy without the addition of small amounts of fish, milk, egg, or even meat. These are sometimes eaten willy-nilly in cake mixes and cooked dishes. Aileen recovered with her former diet that included the herbal remedies for megaloblastic anemia, comfrey and Icelandic moss—both of which contain B-12. In addition, she also ate some cheese, egg, and fish.

ADDITIONAL DIETARY RECOMMENDATIONS

Herbalists recommend the following additions to the diet for both iron-deficient and B-12-deficient anemias:

↩ Dandelion coffee (obtainable in dried form at health-food stores)

↩ Molasses

↩ Desiccated or fresh calf's liver

↩ Cider vinegar, two to three teaspoons in water between meals. This helps to compensate for the shortage of stomach acid that characterizes pernicious anemia

Afterword

"Tired all the time," sometimes referred to in certain medical circles as TATT, is one of the most frequent, most pervasive complaints made by women all over the world, regardless of color, age, and social status. Paradoxically, it is just as likely among the well-to-do and privileged as in areas of poverty and deprivation. It creeps up on its victims gradually, creating increasingly profound mental and physical fatigue for which there is no obvious cause. Sleep and rest give no relief and the sufferer wakes unrefreshed. Today we might say that TATT is related, in some cases, to the condition of CFS, chronic fatigue syndrome.

TATT is often written off by friends, partners, and medics as a trivial neurotic complaint or as minor symptoms of a mental condition such as depression. This may be the explanation in a few cases, but it is more likely that there is a physical condition to account for the lethargy, weakness, inability to relax, and lack of concentration. The mind and body may be struggling against a shortfall in oxygen—this is how it feels—the essential effect of anemia. Nearly a billion women suffer from this insidious disease.

One clue to causation, which is in itself a conundrum, is that a lack of iron occurs more frequently than any other specific nutritional shortage, although it is the second most abundant metal in the earth's crust. The fact that vegetarianism is often seen as trendy in our culture is much to blame, as most vegetarians are wealthy and/or well educated and can choose to eat differently. The poor, on the other hand, have it forced upon them, since meat, the richest source of easily absorbable iron, is expensive.

It is the magic molecule, hemoglobin, in the red corpuscles of the blood, that delivers life-giving oxygen to every part of the body, from brain tissue to toenails. The bottom line: If your spirits are flat, your muscles are slack, and everything is an effort, think ANEMIA—and get a checkup.

Bibliography

Davies, J. *Anemia: A Guide to Causes, Treatment and Prevention.* New York: Harper Collins, 1994.

Davies, J. *Recipes for Health: Anaemia: Over 100 Recipes for Overcoming Iron-Deficiency.* London: Thorsons, 1995.

Demaeyer, E. M. *Preventing and Controlling Iron Deficiency Anaemia Through Primary Health Care: A Guide for Health Administrators and Programme Managers.* Geneva, Switzerland: World Health Organization, 1989.

Eastham, R. D. *Clinical Haematology,* 7th edition. Boston, MA: Butterworth-Heineman, 1992.

Edwards, C. R. W., and I. A. D. Bouchier (eds.). *Davidson's Principles and Practice of Medicine,* 16th edition. New York: Churchill Livingstone, 1991.

Ludlam, C. A. *Clinical Haematology.* New York: Churchill Livingstone, 1990.

Provan, A., and J. Gribben. *Molecular Haematology.* Malden, MA: Blackwell Science Inc., February 2000.

Provan, A. *ABC of Clinical Haematology,* 2nd edition. London: BMJ books, 2002.

Singer, C. R. J., et al. *Oxford Handbook of Clinical Haematology.* New York: Oxford University Press, 1998.

Truswell, A. S. *ABC of Nutrition,* 3rd edition. London: BMJ books, 1999.

Vann Jones, S., and C. R. V. Thomson (eds.). *Essential Medicine* 2nd edition. New York: Churchill Livingstone, 1998.

Websites with other anemia books:

www.geometry.net/health_conditions_bk/anemia.html

www.healthlinkusa.com/bookpage/16_1.html

Resources

UNITED STATES OF AMERICA

Aplastic Anemia Foundation of America/
Aplastic Anemia and MDS International Foundation, Inc.
PO Box 613
Annapolis MD 21404
(800) 747-2820
(410) 867-0242
Fax: (410) 867-0240
E-mail: aamdsoffice@aol.com
Website: http://aamds.org

Iron Disorders Institute Inc.
PO Box 2031
Greenville SC 29602
(888) 565-IRON (4766)
(864) 292-1175
Fax: (864) 292-1878
E-mail: irondis@aol.com
Website: www.irondisorders.org

National Organization for Rare Disorders
55 Kenosia Ave.
PO Box 1968
Danbury CT 06813-1968
(800) 999-6673 (voicemail only)
(203) 744-0100
Fax: (203) 798-2291
E-mail: orphan@rarediseases.org
Website: www.rarediseases.org

National Heart, Lung, and Blood Institute (NHLBI)
PO Box 30105
Bethesda MD 20824-0105
(301) 592-8573
Fax: (301) 592-8563
E-mail: NHLBIinfo@rover.nhlbi.nih.gov
Website: www.nhlbi.nih.gov

CANADA

Anemia Institute for Research and Education
151 Bloor St. West, Ste. 600
Toronto, Ontario M5S 1S4
(877) 99-ANEMIA (in Canada)
(416) 969-7431
Fax: (416) 969-7420
Website: www.anemiainstitute.org

ONLINE COMMUNITIES/ MESSAGE BOARDS

www.mdadvice.com
MDAdvice.com features moderated message boards on many
health topics, including anemia. Unregistered users may read messages, but registration (which is free) is required to post messages.

Index

blood loss, 43; acute, 29, 46, 100; chronic, 30, 46–48, 142–143; and iron deficiency, 43–48

blood tests. *See* tests

blood transfusions, for aplastic anemia, 85; for folate-deficiency anemia, 79; for iron deficiency, 51; for pernicious anemia, 60, 70; for vitamin B-12 deficiency, 60

body mass index (BMI), 99

bone marrow, 17, 19, 21, 33; transplant, 85, 101

breast feeding, 44; vs. bottle feeding, 88–90; and diet, 91–93; guidelines, 90–93; and iron deficiency, 9; and weaning, 93–95

Browning, Elizabeth Barrett, 1

bulimia nervosa, 98–100

C

caffeine, and breast feeding, 91

calcium, and menopause, 123–124; and pregnancy, 109

calorie requirements, 147

cancer, and menopause, 124

captopril, 144

carbimazole, 144

Castle, William, 64

celiac disease, 58, 74

childbirth, 44; and iron deficiency, 10

children, and iron deficiency, 9, 40–42; and iron supplements, 50; and nutrition, 88–95, 148; protein requirements, 20; and vitamin B-12 deficiency, 21

chlorosis, 34

chlorpromazine, 144

chlorpropamide, 144

cigarettes. *See* tobacco

clozapine, 144

cobalamin. *See* vitamin B-12 (cobalamin)

cobalt, 22

constipation, 112

contraceptives, oral, 144

copper, 22

corpuscles, red, 14–16, 21, 30

corpuscles, white, 16

Crohn's disease, 4, 10, 58, 74, 78

D

dapsone, 144

dermatomyositis, 66

diabetes, 59, 66; and menopause, 124

diagnosis, of anemia, 2, 6, 24–32; of iron deficiency, 35–43. *See also* tests

Dictionary of Medicine, 125

diet, 12–13, 48; in adolescence, 97–100; and anemia prevention, 140–141, 145–147; and children, 88–95, 148; importance of, 88; and iron deficiency, 19, 43, 48; and menopause, 119; and natural supplements, 154

diuretics, 60, 76, 78

diverticulitis, 47, 57–58, 117

DNA, 21

dothiepin, 144

dyspareunia, 122

E

eating disorders, 98–100

Elizabeth (Queen Mother), 1, 10, 128, 129

endometriosis, 122

estrogen, 118, 119

exercise, in adolescence, 98; and anemia, 45

extrinsic factor, 64, 70

F

fatigue, 27, 35–36, 67, 117, 145

ferritin, 19

ferrous fumarate, 50

ferrous gluconate, 50

fertility, and menopause, 122–123; and perimenopause, 118; and smoking, 116

fibroid cysts, 4, 10, 121–122

fingernails, 29, 37–38

Floradix herbal iron, 151

folate. *See* folic acid (folate)

folate deficiency anemia, 73–83; and alcohol, 75–77; causes, 73–78; and diet, 73; and heart disorders, 77; and hemolytic anemia, 78; and hypothyroidism, 77; and kidney disease, 77; and pregnancy, 74, 80–81; prevention, 80–83, 131, 139–140; symptoms, 78–79; tests, 79; treatment, 79–80

folic acid (folate), 22, 53, 57, 72–73; and anemia prevention, 80–83, 131, 139–140; and breast feeding, 93; food sources, 82–83, 107; and pregnancy, 74, 80–81, 106–107; requirements, 81

foods, containing folic acid, 82–83, 140; containing iron, 20, 48, 108–109, 139; containing protein, 137–138; containing vitamin C, 140

frusemide, 60

G

gastritis, 58

Glucophage, 59, 62, 144

greensickness, 34

H

hair, 6, 37–38

heart palpitations, 25, 27, 35

heartburn, 112

heme iron, 49, 120, 139

heme molecule, 19

hemoglobin, 1, 19, 20, 130, 155; and aging, 132; and iron, 33; normal levels, 50; and pregnancy, 108; production of, 52; and protein, 136; shortage of, 24; and tobacco, 23

hemoglobinuria, 47

hemolysis, 47

hemolytic anemia, 78

hemorrhoids, 10, 30, 46, 129

herbal medicines, 50, 149–154; and iron-deficiency anemia, 150–153; and vitamin B-12 deficiency, 153–154

heredity, 143

hernia, 46

hydroxocobalamin (vitamin B-12), 61, 70, 71

hyperemesis gravidarum, 112

hyperthyroidism, 22, 66

hypothyroidism, 22, 32, 66; and folate deficiency, 77; and menopause, 124

hysterectomy, 121–122

I

ibuprofen, 10, 144

infection, 17; and pregnancy, 113

inflammatory bowel disorder, 10

inhibin, 118

injections, hydroxocobalamin, 61, 70, 71

ANDROGEN DISORDERS IN WOMEN: The Most Neglected Hormone Problem *by* Theresa Cheung

One in ten women in the U.S. suffers from a disorder caused by an imbalance of the so-called male hormones known as androgens. Symptoms may include facial or body hair growth or loss, dull skin, fatigue, and weight gain.

Because doctors tend to dismiss or ignore such symptoms, there has been little information available on androgen disorders—until now. This book discusses the medical and emotional effects that excessive androgens can have, and outlines the various forms of conventional and alternative treatments.

208 pages ... Paperback $13.95 ... Hardcover $23.95

HOW WOMEN CAN *FINALLY* STOP SMOKING
by Robert C. Klesges, Ph.D., and Margaret DeBon

This guide reveals that what works for men does not necessarily work for women when it comes to quitting smoking. Women tend to gain more weight, their menstrual cycles and menopause affect the likelihood of success, and their withdrawal symptoms are different.

The book is in two parts. *Part One* guides women in choosing the best time to quit and in deciding which method to use. *Part Two* gives directions for managing withdrawal and weight gain, finding peer support, and controlling stress.

192 pages ... 3 illus. ... Paperback $11.95

ONCE A MONTH: Understanding and Treating PMS
by Katharina Dalton, M.D., with Wendy Holton — Revised 6th Edition

Once considered an imaginary complaint, PMS began to receive the serious attention it deserves thanks largely to the work of Katharina Dalton, M.D. Originally written in 1978, this book introduces a whole new genertion to PMS. Fully one-third of the material is new in this sixth edition, from the latest research on how PMS affects learning to the PMS/menopause connection.

Most importantly, Dr. Dalton addresses the whole range of possible treatments—from self-care methods such as the three-hourly starch diet and relaxation techniques to the newest medical options, including updated guidelines for progesterone therapy.

320 pages ... 55 illus. ... Paperback $15.95 ... Hardcover $25.95

All prices subject to change

MENOPAUSE WITHOUT MEDICINE
by Linda Ojeda, Ph.D. ... New Fourth Edition

Linda Ojeda broke new ground 15 years ago with this best-selling resource on menopause, giving women a clear understanding of menopausal changes as well as guidelines for effective self-care.

In this new edition she reexamines the hormone therapy debate; suggests natural remedies for depression, hot flashes, sexual changes, and skin and hair problems; and presents an illustrated basic exercise program. She also includes up-to-date information on natural sources of estrogen, including phytoestrogens, and how diet and personality affect mood swings.

352 pages ... 32 illus. ... 62 tables ... Paperback $15.95 ... Hardcover $25.95

THE NATURAL ESTROGEN DIET: Healthy Recipes for Perimenopause and Menopause
by Dr. Lana Liew with Linda Ojeda, Ph.D.

Two women's health and nutrition experts offer women almost 100 easy and delicious recipes that will naturally increase their estrogen levels. Each recipe includes nutritional information, such as the total calorie, cholesterol, and calcium contents. The authors also provide an overview of how estrogen can be derived from the food we eat, describe which foods are the highest in estrogen content, and offer meal-plan ideas.

224 pages ... 25 illus. ... Paperback $13.95

HER HEALTHY HEART: A Woman's Guide to Preventing and Reversing Heart Disease *Naturally*
by Linda Ojeda, Ph.D.

Almost twice as many women die from heart disease and stroke as from all forms of cancer combined. In fact, heart disease is the #1 killer of American women ages 44 to 65, yet until now most of the research and attention has been directed at men. This book fills this gap by addressing the unique aspects of heart disease in women and the natural ways to prevent it, whether they take hormone replacement therapy (HRT) or not. Ojeda provides detailed information on how to reduce the risk of heart disease through changes in nutrition and diet, physical activity, and stress management.

352 pages ... Paperback $14.95 ... Hardcover $24.95

CHRONIC FATIGUE SYNDROME, FIBROMYALGIA, AND OTHER INVISIBLE ILLNESSES: A Comprehensive and Compassionate Guide *by* Katrina Berne, Ph.D.

A new edition of the classic work *Running on Empty,* this greatly revised and expanded book has the latest findings on chronic fatigue syndrome and comprehensive information about fibromyalgia, a related condition. Overlapping diseases such as environmental illness, breast implant inflammatory syndrome, lupus, Sjögren's syndrome, and post-polio syndrome are also discussed. The book includes possible causes, symptoms, diagnostic processes, and options for treatment.

400 pages ... Paperback $15.95 ... Hardcover $25.95

THE ART OF GETTING WELL: A Five-Step Plan for Maximizing Health When You Have a Chronic Illness *by* David Spero, R.N., Foreword by Martin L. Rossman, M.D.

Self-management programs have become a key way for people to deal with chronic illness. In this book, David Spero brings together the medical, psychological, and spiritual aspects of getting well in a five-step approach: slow down and use your energy for the things and people that matter — make small, progressive changes that build self-confidence — get help and nourish the social ties that are crucial for well-being — value your body and treat it with affection and respect — take responsibility for getting the best care and health you can.

224 pages ... Paperback $15.95 ... Hardcover $25.95

CHINESE HERBAL MEDICINE MADE EASY: Natural and Effective Remedies for Common Illnesses *by* Thomas Richard Joiner

Chinese herbal medicine is an ancient system for maintaining health and prolonging life. This book demystifies the subject, by providing clear explanations and easy-to-read alphabetical listings of more than 750 herbal remedies for over 250 common illnesses ranging from acid reflux and AIDS to breast cancer, pain management, sexual dysfunction, and weight loss. Whether you are a newcomer to herbology or a seasoned practitioner, you will find this book to be a valuable addition to your health library.

432 pages ... Paperback $24.95 ... Hardcover $34.95

Order from our website at www.hunterhouse.com

ORDER FORM

10% DISCOUNT on orders of $50 or more —
20% DISCOUNT on orders of $150 or more —
30% DISCOUNT on orders of $500 or more —
On cost of books for fully prepaid orders

NAME

ADDRESS

CITY/STATE   ZIP/POSTCODE

PHONE   COUNTRY (outside of U.S.)

TITLE	QTY	PRICE	TOTAL
Anemia in Women (paperback)		@ $12.95	

Prices subject to change without notice

Please list other titles below:

		@ $	
		@ $	
		@ $	
		@ $	
		@ $	
		@ $	
		@ $	
		@ $	

Check here to receive our book catalog ☐   free

Shipping Costs

By Priority Mail: first book $4.50, each additional book $1.00
By UPS and to Canada: first book $5.50, each additional book $1.50
For rush orders and other countries call us at (510) 865-5282

TOTAL	_____
Less discount @____%	(_____)
TOTAL COST OF BOOKS	_____
Calif. residents add sales tax	_____
Shipping & handling	_____
TOTAL ENCLOSED	_____
Please pay in U.S. funds only	

☐ Check ☐ Money Order ☐ Visa ☐ MasterCard ☐ Discover

Card # _____ Exp. date _____

Signature _____

Complete and mail to:
Hunter House Inc., Publishers
PO Box 2914, Alameda CA 94501-0914
Website: www.hunterhouse.com
Orders: (800) 266-5592 or email: ordering@hunterhouse.com
Phone (510) 865-5282   Fax (510) 865-4295

AIW — 9/2002